Translating Chronic Illness Research into Practice

Edited by

Debbie Kralik PhD, RN
Barbara Paterson PhD, RN
Vivien Coates PhD, RN

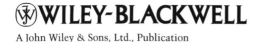
WILEY-BLACKWELL
A John Wiley & Sons, Ltd., Publication

Blackwell Publishing was acquired by John Wiley & Sons in February 2007. Blackwell's publishing programme has been merged with Wiley's global Scientific, Technical, and Medical business to form Wiley-Blackwell.

Registered office
John Wiley & Sons Ltd, The Atrium, Southern Gate, Chichester, West Sussex, PO19 8SQ, United Kingdom

Editorial offices
9600 Garsington Road, Oxford, OX4 2DQ, United Kingdom
2121 State Avenue, Ames, Iowa 50014-8300, USA

For details of our global editorial offices, for customer services and for information about how to apply for permission to reuse the copyright material in this book please see our website at www.wiley.com/wiley-blackwell.

Library of Congress Cataloging-in-Publication Data

Translating chronic illness research into practice / edited by Debbie Kralik, Barbara Paterson, Vivien Coates.
      p. ; cm.
   Includes bibliographical references and index.
   ISBN 978-1-4051-5965-4 (pbk. : alk. paper) 1. Chronic diseases. 2. Chronic diseases – Research.
I. Kralik, Debbie. II. Paterson, Barbara L. III. Coates, Vivien E. (Vivien Elizabeth), 1957–
   [DNLM: 1. Chronic Disease – Review. 2. Biomedical Research – Review. WT 500 T772 2010]
   RA644.5.T73 2010
   616′.044 – dc22
                                                                                    2009040325

A catalogue record for this book is available from the British Library.

Set in 9.5/11.5 pt Palatino by Laserwords Private Limited, Chennai, India

Printed in the UK

Contents

Contents

List of Contributors

Celeste Alvaro, *PhD.* Post-Doctoral Fellow and Project Coordinator, Health Promotion Research Centre, Dalhousie University, Halifax, Nova Scotia, Canada

Malcolm Battersby, *PhD, FRANZCP, FAChAM, MBBS.* Associate Professor and Director, Flinders Human Behaviour and Health Research Unit, Flinders University, Adelaide, South Australia

Alastair Buchan, Professor, University of Oxford (incoming Dean of Medicine), and Acute Stroke Programme, Nuffield Department of Medicine, John Radcliffe Hospital, Oxford, UK

Vivien Coates, *PhD, RN.* Professor of Nursing Research, School of Nursing, University of Ulster, Coleraine, County Londonderry, UK. Assistant Director of Nursing (R&D) Western Health and Social Care Trust, Trust Headquarters, Londonderry, UK

Max Hopwood, *PhD, BA (Hons).* Research Fellow, National Centre in HIV Social Research, The University of New South Wales, New South Wales, Australia

Marit Kirkevold, Professor of Nursing Science, University of Oslo, Oslo, Norway

Alison Kitson, *PhD, RN, FRCN.* Fellow, Green College, University of Oxford, Oxford, UK

Debbie Kralik, *PhD, RN.* General Manager, Strategy and Research, Royal District Nursing Service, South Australia, and Associate Professor, University of South Australia and Adelaide University, South Australia

Sharon Lawn, *PhD, MSW, DipEd, BA.* Researcher, Flinders Human Behaviour and Health Research Unit, and Senior Lecturer, Flinders University, School of Medicine, Department of Psychiatry, Adelaide, South Australia

Antonia van Loon, *PhD, RN.* Senior Research Fellow, Royal District Nursing Service, South Australia, and Adjunct Faculty, Flinders University, Adelaide, South Australia

Renee F. Lyons, *PhD.* Tier 1, Canada Research Chair in Health Promotion. Professor, School of Health and Human Performance, Department of Psychology, and School of Nursing, Dalhousie University. Senior Scientist, Atlantic Health Promotion Research Centre, Halifax, Nova Scotia, Canada

Lynn McIntyre, *MD, MHSc, FRCPC.* Professor and CIHR Chair in Gender and Health, Department of Community Health Sciences, Faculty of Medicine, University of Calgary, Alberta, Canada

David B. Nicholas, *PhD.* The Hospital for Sick Children, Toronto, Ontario, Canada

Barbara Paterson, *PhD, RN.* Professor and Tier 1 Canada Research Chair in Chronic Illness, Faculty of Nursing, University of New Brunswick, Canada

Rene Pols, *FRANZCP, FAFPHM, MBBS.* Deputy Director, Flinders Human Behaviour and Health Research Unit. Senior Lecturer, Flinders University, School of Medicine, Department of Psychiatry, Adelaide. Consultant Psychiatrist, Southern Mental Health, Adelaide, South Australia

Ian Reckless, Consultant Physician, Oxford Biomedical Research Centre, John Radcliffe Hospital, Oxford, UK

Grace Warner, *PhD.* Assistant Professor, School of Occupational Therapy, Dalhousie University, Halifax, Nova Scotia, Canada

Sally Wellard, *PhD, RN.* Professor of Nursing, School of Nursing, University of Ballarat, Victoria, Australia

Allison Williams, *PhD, RN.* Postdoctoral Research Fellow, School of Nursing, The University of Melbourne, Victoria, Australia

Preface

The purpose of this book is to provide both a synthesis and a critique of recent advances in chronic illness research and to consider the applicability of that research to chronic illness prevention, treatment and care. The aim has been to present an overview of recent chronic illness research and to profile examples of the applications of such research in clinical practice.

Health care does not occur in a vacuum, but is intrinsically linked to politics, environment, culture and society. Globally, it is a fact that no country will have sufficient resources to address completely the health-care wants and needs of its people. Increasingly, we need to think globally but act locally using the best evidence available as an indicator of effective care intervention. Researchers and practitioners alike are aware that if research is to inform chronic illness prevention, treatment and care, it must be studied in ways that acknowledge the complexity of the chronic illness experience and transcend the boundaries of the relationship between the person with the illness and the health-care provider. Provided in this book are detailed examples in which interdisciplinary, transdisciplinary and multidisciplinary teams of researchers have developed initiatives that have been successful in assisting people with chronic illness to live well. However, many of these initiatives may be unknown to health-care practitioners who have confined their reading of research-based evidence to journals and texts in their own language, discipline and/or nation. The editors of this book have brought together internationally renowned researchers in chronic illnesses to present an overview of recent advances and to suggest future directions in chronic illness research, prevention, treatment and care.

To achieve the purpose of translating chronic illness research into practice, we focus on the key concepts of chronic illness, practice, research on chronic illness and translating research into practice. Within the book, several authors define chronic illness as they have interpreted it for their chapters. The concepts of translation and practice are defined as follows: 'Translation research transforms currently available knowledge into useful measures for everyday clinical and public health practice' (Narayan *et al.* 2004, p. 959).

The gap between research and practice is well recognised and this book illuminates some of the complexities of applying evidence to practice, and through these discussions aims to make a contribution to bridging this gap and thus is a resource to others wishing to underpin their practice with research. 'Practice' refers to the integration of knowledge and/or theory about health promotion, chronic disease prevention, the management of chronic illness or the experience of living with chronic illness in the performance of a clinical, research or policy development role. A wide range of research that is of relevance to chronic illness has been presented and authors have either provided a critique or an interpretation of its potential utility or limitations for application to practice. In this way, this book is making relevant research available to users and also illustrating how it might be, or indeed has already been, used in the fields of health promotion, clinical management or policy making.

Chapter 1 sets the scene by developing our understanding of chronic illness research globally, and then serves to identify barriers and enablers to advancing knowledge about prevention and management of chronic illnesses. The need is identified for a universal understanding of the chronic disease experience that goes beyond the biomedical perspective to build a stronger foundation for health promotion and disease prevention initiatives.

Transition, as a chronic illness experience, is the focus of Chapter 2. An overview of the different conceptualisations of transition is provided, detailing areas of ambiguity in the research. A transition framework relevant for health practice when working with people with chronic illness is detailed.

Chapter 3 explores the translation of chronic illness research across the lifespan of a person. It highlights the relevance of a developmental perspective on chronic illness in order to understand how chronic illness and human development interact to impact on the life of individuals and families across the lifespan. A review is provided of central tenets of the human development perspective, followed by a brief review of the current state of affairs with regard to applying a lifespan developmental perspective in chronic illness research. Finally, examples of chronic illness research informed by a lifespan developmental perspective are reviewed.

Chapter 4 provides an overview of how co-morbidity has been conceptualised within the various health-care disciplines, which has contributed to the frag-mentation, replication and omissions in care of people with co-morbidities. The inequities in health care and the influences of the social determinants of how people with co-morbidity respond to and manage their health are also discussed. The debate about how best to manage multiple chronic illnesses from the vari-ous stakeholders is highlighted, drawing attention to the need for longitudinal approaches to health-care delivery to ensure continuity of care.

The international, historical and policy contexts of self-management are explored in Chapter 5. Concepts are described, which overlap with or inform an understanding of self-management from both the person's perspective and the health professional's perspective. This chapter also broadens our understandings of self-management concepts and practical applications of these.

Chapter 6 is a synthesis of published international research about self-management interventions within the field of type 2 diabetes. It presents a critical view of the self-management education and/or behavioural support inter-ventions that have been reported in the published literature for the purpose of revealing how the way the interventions have been framed by researchers has influenced who chooses to participate and to remain in the intervention.

The focus of Chapter 7 is the emergence of technology for supporting patients and their families. An overview of research is provided regarding the use and outcomes of technology in fostering the self-management of chronic illness, including locating and discussing gaps and areas of ambiguity in current work.

Finally, Chapter 8 looks to the future of chronic illness and chronic illness research. It explores how we might positively modify future projections of chronic illness by building upon the revolution that is happening in some parts of the globe in knowledge translation.

Practitioners and researchers across the globe have much to learn from each other and enhancing this communication would benefit all parties. The growing burden of chronic illness – both communicable and non-communicable – across the world and creative responses by researchers in various disciplines to those challenges can provide important lessons (and research opportunities). This book is intended as a text and resource for researchers and practitioners across health disciplines as well as for graduate students within the health professions and the social sciences. It will also inform academic researchers, government policy experts, health plan and consumer representatives regarding available research in the field.

We anticipate that this book will contribute to the dialogue and debate that focus on and explicate our knowledge and the different ways of knowing in chronic illness research and practice. It has been a privlege to work with the contributing authors and to experience their commitment to the care and well-being of people living with chronic illness.

Debbie Kralik
Barbara Paterson
Vivien Coates

Reference

Narayan, K.M.V., Benjamin, E., Gregg, E.W., Norris, S.L., Engelgau, M.M. (2004) Diabetes translation research: where are we and where do we want to be? *Annals of Internal Medicine* **140**(11): 958–964.

1. Globalisation of Chronic Illness Research

Sally Wellard

Introduction

This chapter builds on my previous work (Wellard 1998) where I have explored discursive constructions of chronic illness and argued that discourses of science, individualism and normalisation underpinned our ways of working with people experiencing chronic illnesses and the research questions that are posed. The aims of this chapter are (a) to develop a contemporary understanding of chronic illness research globally and (b) to identify barriers and enablers to advancing knowledge about prevention and management of chronic illnesses.

A review of contemporary literature identified a number of significant shifts that are relevant to the aims of this chapter, most notably the recognition of chronic illnesses as an urgent problem affecting global health. Discourses of science remain evident, but an increasing emphasis on economic and social consequences of chronic illnesses is emerging. There are a number of challenges in attempting to gain a global view of work in the field of chronic illness. First, the literature surrounding chronic illness is vast and the volume of material is overwhelming. Second, the analysis presented in this chapter is limited by my reliance on the English language. Although there is considerable work related to chronic illness published in many other languages, it was not accessible to me. Third, there are limitations in the databases available for bibliometric analysis by researchers. For example, Hofman *et al.* (2006) identified that MEDLINE 'does not equally represent all countries, journals or topics' (p. 418), resulting in a poor or inaccurate representation of research in middle- and low-income countries.

The strategy adopted for developing a contemporary view of the globalisation of chronic illness work was to develop an integrative literature review with the goal of developing a critical analytical view of trends in the field. GOOGLE scholar (http://scholar.google.com/) and MEDLINE database (using PubMed: http://www.ncbi.nlm.nih.gov/sites/entrez/) were searched, identifying the range of literature published between 1995 and 2007. Additionally, a search of the World Health Organization (WHO) web pages (http://www.who.int/en/)

1

revealed relevant reports and links. The main search terms used were chronic illness, chronic disease, research, management and prevention. References in recently published work were scrutinised, and textbooks were hand searched.

What is in a name?

The first striking feature in reviewing recent literature related to chronic illnesses is the variety of terms that are frequently used as synonyms for chronic illness with little acknowledgement of the meanings implied in their use. Predominant terms identified included chronic illness (CI), chronic disease (CD), chronic conditions (CC), non-communicable disease (NCD) and chronic illness and disability (CID). Terminology matters, and the absence of a clear definition can blur meanings and assumptions inherent in the arguments presented by authors. Gerber *et al.* (2007) also noted the scarcity of a conceptual definition of disease and illness, raising concerns about adopting recommendations from research without understanding the premises on which such investigations are based.

The interchangeable use of the terms *disease* and *illness* is not new. Larsen (2006) argued that differentiation between these terms is important. Disease refers to the practitioner's view of pathophysiological alterations in a person's condition, associated with an objective medical view of a human ailment (Hofmann 2002) and the assignment of a diagnosis (Wikman *et al.* 2005). Illness, however, refers to the perceived human experience of living with and responding to disease by those with the disease and the people who live with them (Taylor 2005; Larsen 2006). Illness is frequently referred to as a subjective interpretation of disease (Hofmann 2002). These terms are broad and imprecise (Wikman *et al.* 2005); they could refer to minor conditions with low impact or very serious conditions with life-limiting effects.

The concept of chronicity, most simply defined, relates to the temporality of a condition where changes in health are ongoing and will not be cured by a short course of treatment or surgery (Miller 2000). Various publications attempt to create more specific detail, but there remains little consensus around a more precise definition. Some authors indicate that a chronic illness must have a duration of more than 6 months (O'Halloran *et al.* 2003), whereas others are less specific, with greater focus on the ongoing nature of illness and the accompanying complexity and adjustment in daily life as criteria denoting chronicity (Price 1996).

The terms *chronic disease* and *chronic illness* remain the most commonly used. Another term found in the psychological literature, *chronic illness and disability* (CID), is of interest in this discussion because it assumes a coupling of illness and disability (Livneh 2001). Livneh and Antonak (2005), rather than defining CID, list characteristics commonly associated with CID to include some functional limitations and an effect on capacity to carry out daily activities; uncertain prognosis and a long-term need for medical and rehabilitative care; experience of psychosocial stress related to the condition; impact on family; and sustained financial loss (p. 12). This definition would exclude some common chronic ailments, such as hypertension, where there is often little or no impact on daily activities.

The recent emergence of new terminology appears to be an attempt to create an umbrella term that will be inclusive of the different understandings of chronic ailments and link different audiences to look more at the overarching issues related to chronicity in the world. For example, the term *chronic conditions* (CC) now frequently appears in Australian literature, used by the federal government agencies, and is often used interchangeably with chronic disease. For example, O'Halloran *et al.* (2003), in a report for the Australian Institute of Health and Welfare, defined chronic conditions as those lasting at least 6 months, showing a pattern of deterioration or periods of relapse and remission, having a poor prognosis or possible lack of curability and disease-related effects, including co-morbid conditions. The use of the word *condition* is increasingly visible in programmes that engage different stakeholders (consumers, health-care professionals and educationalists) who are sponsored by the Australian Department of Health and Ageing.

The term *non-communicable disease* (NCD) appears in many publications related to international discussion across a number of sectors (e.g. the WHO, United Nations and World Bank). Although the term is increasingly used in literature, there remains little definition and an implicit assumption that these terms are commonly understood. Non-communicable disease does focus attention away from infectious diseases but remains contentious as a descriptor for chronic illness/disease because some infectious diseases can also be chronic (e.g. malaria).

In this chapter, the term *chronic illness* has been adopted to refer to ongoing alteration in health, except where I am specifically addressing a particular disease or group of diseases, or representing the arguments of others.

Global crisis in chronic illness

Until recently, popular understandings of global health were dichotomised. Chronic illnesses were generally portrayed as ailments of the populations of developed countries (e.g. heart disease, diabetes and cancer) and associated with affluent lifestyles leading to increased risks linked with energy-dense high-fat diets and inactivity. Conversely, infectious diseases were largely portrayed as ailments of developing countries (e.g. bacterial and viral diarrhoeal diseases) associated with poverty and insufficient infrastructure to prevent their spread. The United Nations Millennium development goals adopted in 2000 reflect that dichotomised view, with a focus on addressing factors that will reduce the incidence of infectious diseases (more details of the goals are available at http://www.un.org/millenniumgoals/).

This dichotomised view has recently been challenged with increased attention to what is argued by many as a global epidemic of chronic disease (Horton 2005). The WHO estimates that death from chronic diseases in 2005 is double the death rate from the combined causes of infectious diseases, perinatal and maternal conditions and nutritional deficiencies (WHO 2005). The global distribution of mortality from chronic illness has significantly changed, with 80% of deaths from chronic illnesses now occurring in low- and middle-income countries (Strong *et al.* 2006).

The change in prevalence of chronic illness has been associated with the increasing ageing of the world's population. Strong *et al.* (2005) estimated that 'all chronic diseases account for 72% of the total global burden of disease in the population aged 30 years and over' (p. 1579). This represents a significant burden not only for individuals and their families but also high economic and social costs for countries (WHO 2005). The *WHO Global Report* (2005) identified cardiovascular diseases, cancer, chronic respiratory diseases and diabetes as the leading contributing factors to the chronic illness epidemic. In many low- and middle-income countries, these diseases occur more commonly in younger adults than in high-income countries and result in earlier mortality. Chronic illness does not exist only among adults; there has been a worldwide increase in childhood obesity in the past decade in low-, middle- and high-income countries, with an associated rise in the prevalence of type 2 diabetes in children and adolescents (WHO 2005).

The risk factors of many chronic illnesses are well known. They are considered modifiable and include unhealthy diet, physical inactivity and the use of tobacco (WHO 2005). However, these risk factors associated with lifestyle are complex to address. Strong *et al.* (2005) argue against the common myth that unhealthy behaviours are related to poor choice of individuals, directing attention to the interplay of environment, economy and increasing urbanisation being influential in poor diet and limited access to activity in low- and middle-income countries. The influence and impact of chronic illness differs across the globe and similarly the emphasis in research differs.

Impact of chronic illness in developing nations

Research related to chronic illness in developing countries (low and middle income) has a strong emphasis on measuring the prevalence and impact of chronic illness, using mortality and disability-adjusted life years (DALYs) as indicators of the burden of disease (Strong *et al.* 2005). The growth in population-based health surveillance studies has facilitated a commensurate growth in research, expanding knowledge and understanding about the social determinants of health.

The investigation of the burden of disease has been undertaken for many decades, but has recently received greater prominence with the development of more sophisticated methodologies and improved access to data sets, facilitating a global analysis of information at the population level. It is now possible to link incidence of disease with both short-term and long-term health outcomes and with mortality (Mathers *et al.* 2001). Morbidity is assessed using DALYs, where 'one DALY can be thought of as one lost year of healthy life and the burden of disease as a measurement of the gap between current health of a population and an ideal situation where everyone lives to old age in full health' (Strong *et al.* 2005, p. 1579). The Global Burden of Disease study (WHO 2005) now represents analysis across a greater number of low- and middle-income countries with more detail, including information relating to educational levels. This global study provides baseline data from which effectiveness of interventions can be evaluated and further analysis of changes in distribution of mortality and burden of disease across countries can be made.

The goal of this chapter is not to discuss the status of any specific chronic illness; however, the level of obesity in low- and middle-income countries is striking and therefore will be briefly presented. Prentice (2006) reviewed the epidemiological data on obesity and reports that the obesity 'pandemic is penetrating the poorest nations in the world – first amongst the urban middle-aged adults, but increasingly affecting semi-urban and rural areas, and younger age groups' (p. 93). His examination of Gambia as a case study revealed significant differences in rates of obesity within the country, although the overall rate of obesity for the country was relatively low at 4%. Women were significantly more obese than men, with 32% of women over 30 years being obese, compared to less than 2% of males. Additionally, obesity was higher in urban-dwelling people. While childhood malnutrition remains a concern in developing countries, there is also an emerging incidence of childhood obesity in these countries. Poverty, reduced access to quality foods and limitations on physical activity associated with overcrowded urban developments are considered to be contributing to these changes in childhood obesity (WHO 2005).

There has been rapid expansion in the study of social factors associated with poor health. The seminal work of Doyal and Pennell (1979) exploring the political economy of health demonstrated that ill health is not solely related to medically defined causes, but is a product of inequalities arising from the social and economic organisation of society. In the past decade, considerable research has explored and expanded our understandings of what are now commonly referred to as the *social determinants of health* (Irwin *et al.* 2006). Gross inequalities in health have been identified within and between countries (Marmot 2005). The establishment of the Commission on Social Determinants of Health (a WHO initiative) in 2005 is an active strategy to advance systematic research to reduce health inequities in partnership with individual low- and middle-income countries (Irwin *et al.* 2006).

Poverty and inequity in consumption of resources underpin the social determinants of health (Judson 2004). Poverty is linked to social status, race, gender and education. Wilkinson and Marmot (2003) summarised the social determinants of health into 10 key areas to inform action to address inequities: the social gradient, stress, early life, social exclusion, work, unemployment, social support, addiction, food and transport. Broad-based action, rather than medical-specific action, is clearly indicated to address the social determinants of health. Continuing to invest in medically driven health services without concurrent attention to these factors will have little impact on the overall rates of chronic illness. For example, Le Galès-Camus (2005) argued that banning tobacco advertising and increasing taxes on cigarettes are effective preventative strategies against tobacco-related cardiovascular disease and cancer and are needed in low- and middle-income countries. This type of strategy has a much greater impact on reducing the rate of tobacco-related disease and reduces the subsequent demand for high-cost medical services. Prevention is considerably less expensive than treatment, but systematic

5

preventative health programmes are limited in their effectiveness by inconsistent distribution in many countries.

Trends in chronic illness research in developed nations

Understanding the prevalence and impact of chronic illness remains part of the research agenda in high-income countries; however, given their greater resources, a number of additional areas of research related to chronic illness are prominent. There is now considerable understanding of the sociological aspects of living with chronic illness that has influenced the growth in the work exploring connections between peoples' experience of illness and the ways in which they can be supported in that experience (Taylor & Bury 2007). There is extensive literature about the meaning and significance chronic illnesses have for individuals and their families across a wide variety of diagnoses (e.g. diabetes, renal disease and multiple sclerosis [MS], to name a few). Thorne and Paterson (2000) referred to this area of research as *insider research*, which has included exploration of bodily experiences of illness (Kelly & Field 1996; Wilde 2003), the impact of living with illness on people's social worlds (Livneh 2001) and their experiences of stigma and social exclusion (Wellard & Beddoes 2005; Lubkin & Larsen 2006). There is a clear acknowledgement of the importance of illness narratives to people living with chronic illness (Charmaz 2000; Werner *et al.* 2004).

Personal accounts or narratives of illness experiences have facilitated increased understandings of the multiple ways in which people respond to chronic illness and develop personal approaches to assist them in living with the illness and its effects (Wellard 1998; Mengshoel & Heggen 2004). Hardy (2002) documented the diversity of ways in which narratives are expressed among those with chronic illness, and the way the Internet has been appropriated by many people to extend the form of their narrative expression. The Internet has expanded the available space for narratives, and the use of 'home pages' now provides a dynamic and potentially interactive space for moving beyond accounts of individual experiences to places where people also provide advice and, in some instances, advocate particular approaches to care. It is likely that growth in the provision of advice via the Internet will expand further with 'e-commerce', facilitating increased individual marketing of advice globally (Hardy 2002).

Another focus of recent research has been to understand the transitions that occur in the lives of people with chronic illnesses and how people respond and adapt to these transitions. Kralik *et al.* (2006) argued that transitions involve a change over time where the persons reconstruct their self-identity. Transitions for people with chronic illness are not linear and are differentiated from earlier work on illness trajectories that suggested predictable pathways and stages in disease progression (Wellard 1998). Transitions are triggered by turning point events (Rasmussen *et al.* 2007) and for people with chronic illness, these can be predictable or unpredictable, cyclical and potentially recurring throughout life and result in the persons redeveloping their ways of living with illness (Kralik 2002). In a recent study of young women with diabetes, relationships with people, both social and with health professionals, were found to be important in managing transitions successfully (Rasmussen *et al.* 2007).

The complexity of, and variable quality in, relationships between people with chronic illness and professionals in the health-care system have been widely reported and arguably contribute to a level of difficulty for many in managing their illness (Thorne 2006; Wellard *et al.* 2007). Frequently, health professionals act as gatekeepers of health services, effectively controlling access to resources. This is in part due to a need to ration resources but it is also a reflection of the authoritative power of professional knowledge within our current systems (Clapton & Kendall 2002; Thorne 2006). More recent challenges to the assumption of the health professional being the expert suggest the need to recognise that patients are experts in their own right; this recognition is an important part of building successful partnerships in health-care provision. Fox (2005) summarised the debate in identifying the forms of expertise that both patients and professionals bring to the health-care relationship. Patients have expertise in the specific experience of their illness, their social situation, the levels of risk they are prepared to accept, their own values and preferences for living and treatment choices. Health professionals bring expertise in general understanding of disease (including aetiology, diagnosis and prognosis), the available treatment options, associated risks and probable health outcomes. Both levels of expertise and perceptions of that expertise vary among patients and professionals (Fox 2005).

There has been a shift from the use of the label *patient* when referring to people with chronic illness to the label *consumer* in some literature. There are a number of different constructions of the term *consumer* within the chronic illness field. Consumer groups bring together interested people associated with a specific illness or group of illnesses (including patients, carers and professionals) to provide a public voice about the issues and concerns of the members (Allsop *et al.* 2004). For example, in Australia, the Chronic Illness Alliance has represented over 40 consumer and advocacy groups on matters of common concern to promote the interests of those with chronic illness to the government, health professional groups and health service providers. The MS society is an example of a single illness focus consumer group that lobbies for resources, funds research and provides services specifically to people with MS. Consumer groups like these have the potential to influence policy and services that are more responsive to the needs of people with specific chronic illness.

The term consumer has also been used to refer to those people who use health-care services. The term is associated with a broader change within Western societies where ideologies of privatisation and market predominate (Allen 2007). Increased access to information has led to consumers being well informed and knowledgeable about their rights, including the right to be treated fairly in transactions and the right to purchase and consume what they desire. Consumers of health-care services have also become better informed about medical knowledge and treatment options (Woolf *et al.* 2005). However, Walker (2007) argued that the underpinning assumption that all consumers have equal capacity to choose and participate is fallacious because choices in health consumption are greatly influenced by individual circumstances including income, geographical location and disease severity.

Part of the consumer focus in health care has been the introduction of consumer models of care where partnerships between provider and consumer aim to deliver better outcomes; however, there are a number of impediments to engaging in consumer partnerships in health (Wellard *et al.* 2003; Penney & Wellard 2007). Barriers to engaging in partnerships for care with consumers are diverse and reflect the often experienced gap between espoused ideals and practical realities of health service delivery in a constantly evolving system where innovation frequently outstrips the resources to support it. While recognising the shift towards consumerism, the structures of health-care services continue to position users of services as patients who rely on professional expertise, frequently reconstructing paternalism as a silent foundation for professional practice.

Patient-centred care has been argued to be a cornerstone of health-care practice and identified as a shared value among health professionals where practice is guided by principles of what is 'good' for patients and their families (McGrath *et al.* 2006). Patient-centred care implies that care focuses on the persons as a whole, not only on their disease and symptoms, and therefore it requires partnerships between health-care professionals, patients, their family and caregivers. Partnerships arguably lead to improved health outcomes and increased levels of satisfaction for all stakeholders. However, there is increasing recognition that involving people in partnership for care is highly desired but difficult to deliver (Penney & Wellard 2007). There has been notable growth in the active involvement of consumers at the macro level of health-care services, including consumer roles on boards of management, ethics committees and consumer reference groups. These activities are important and have had some impact on shifting the focus of health-care organisations to consumer needs rather than professional and institutional needs. Wider micro-level partnerships in care are less evident. A recent doctoral work of Penney (2005) identified the struggle of both nurses and older consumers to understand how partnerships in care can occur in the current organisation of health-care services where staff experience constraints in both time and space. The structures of health-care services position consumers with the identity of patient and consequently subject to a range of mechanisms associated with legal and risk management regulations.

Policy drivers: taking action

The global challenge is increasingly clear. There is a need for radical shifts in the way health is managed to address the impact of the epidemic of chronic illness. Clarity about preventable risk factors and optimal disease management provide clear direction for action in the prevention and control of chronic illnesses. The WHO (2005) has developed a detailed evidence-based action plan to assist countries in identifying potential strategies for reducing the burden of chronic illness, which needs to target both populations and individuals and recognise the social determinants of health. Taxation and price control, for example, could make alcohol and tobacco less affordable and provide subsidies to reduce the costs of healthy foods. Similarly, investing in improving the built environment in community-based projects could assist in providing accessible safe spaces for increased activity. These are preventative strategies. Additionally, WHO (2005) makes recommendations for the effective improvement of chronic disease management including the establishment and maintenance of effective clinical information systems, the provision of multidisciplinary health-care teams with an emphasis on primary health care and support for patient self-management programmes. While the arguments in support of these strategies are clear, the feasibility of implementation is more problematic. Implementation of taxation reform and prioritisation of infrastructure development, which lays emphasis on preventative health, are sensitive political issues and in all countries compete with other stakeholders who prioritise economic investment differently. Discussion of the complex socio-political landscape that influences the advancement of these strategies is beyond the scope of this chapter. However, the strategy for promoting patient self-management has received considerable attention and will now be explored.

Self-management has been increasingly adopted as part of health policy in a number of developed countries (e.g. in the UK policy 'Expert Patient: A New Approach to Chronic Illness for the 21st Century' [Fox 2005] and in Australia as part of the Chronic Disease Strategy [Dowrick 2006]). The idea of self-management programmes situates persons with chronic illness as central, with expertise and understanding of their illness and the ability (actual or potential) to assume responsibility of their management of their own health. Self-management programmes also assume some form of partnership between the individuals with the illness, the family, carers and health professionals. Self-management is most commonly conceived as involving:

> ... the individual with a chronic condition working in partnership with their carers and health professionals so that they can: know their condition and various treatment options; negotiate a plan of care; engage in activities that protect and promote health, monitor and manage symptoms and signs of illness, manage the impact of illness on physical functioning, emotions and interpersonal relationships.
>
> (McDonald et al. 2004, p. 1 cited in Beckmann et al. 2007)

There are a number of different approaches to patient self-management, but the most widely adopted model internationally was developed by Kate Lorig and colleagues at Stanford University and based on a self-efficacy approach (Lorig & Holman 2003). The Stanford model uses a peer-led approach with a focus on sustained behavioural change. Advocates of this model have published evidence of demonstrated benefits using the widely accepted methods of randomised trials (Gifford *et al.* 1998; Lorig *et al.* 1999).

Self-management programmes also have critics. Concern has been raised about the focus self-management programmes place on individuals which ignores, or marginalises, the broader social and economic context that influences illness experiences and individual responses to self-care (Kendall & Rogers 2007). The underpinning assumption of locating the control at the individual level dislocates social responsibilities for illness management and places the burden of care on the person with the illness. Self-management programmes, while focused on individuals, are largely sponsored and managed by health-care agencies and therefore threaten the autonomy of individuals to determine their own pathway to care. As Kendall and Rogers (2007) point out, it is difficult for professionals 'because they operate in systems that demand throughput at defined costs, which undermines their capacity to operate in ways that facilitate self-management' (p. 131) and support models promoting compliance with professional advice.

Self-management programmes have been implemented as part of a suite of chronic illness management systems in developed countries. In the United Kingdom, self-management programming is the third tier after case management (intensive management of people with multiple complex conditions) and disease management (focused at people identified as those at risk). Self-management approaches are expected to support people at low risk, anticipated to be 70% of people with chronic illness (Kendall & Rogers 2007). Therefore, as Kendall and Rogers argue, self-management is being promoted as the predominant strategy for chronic illness management and is diminishing the broader social responsibility (and consequently reducing government costs) for care provision.

Global initiatives for future chronic illness management

It becomes evident from exploring selected aspects of chronic illness research across the globe that the impact of chronic illness is complex. There are wide variations, yet significant commonalities, in the prevalence and burden of chronic illnesses. However, there is a tendency for simplification in how chronic illness issues are presented because the complexity is hard to represent. Any approach to advancing chronic illness management needs to integrate population and individual strategies and include prevention and ongoing care and support. While the relative burden of illness and the resources available to support health care in countries vary, a major barrier to developing improved chronic illness care remains, with a strong emphasis on acute health problems in health-care systems (Weeramanthri et al. 2003; Yach et al. 2004).

This emphasis on acute health problems is grounded in the biomedical approach that primarily focuses on disease and remains the core orientation in medical and most health professional education for entry to practice (Tinetti & Fried 2004). Tinetti and Fried (2004) argue that the continued focus on disease and acute problems within a context of increasing chronicity 'inadvertently leads to under treatment, overtreatment, or mistreatment' (p. 179). Under-treatment arises when people present for care with symptoms that do not 'fit' with accepted diagnostic criteria or where interventions are limited to the biological cause of illness rather than also directed at addressing underlying social determinants of illness (e.g. counselling and direction to social support services). Overtreatment has been noted as including over-medication and associated adverse reactions as well as high levels of aggressive disease management in the very old. Mistreatment, Tinetti and Fried (2004) suggest, is inadvertent but occurs nonetheless because treatment is based on disease-based decision-making rather than patient preferences. These consequences of a disease-oriented system, identified by Homer *et al.* (2007) in a system analysis, showed that people who are sick have remained sick because of elements of the system and because of a lack of investment in prevention and early intervention. A disease orientation provides clinicians with more predictable approaches to care with evidence-based guidelines for a wide range of conditions, whereas chronic illness management presents considerably less certainty (Weeramanthri *et al.* 2003) with illness pathways that are highly variable and unpredictable.

Developing different approaches to health-care needs to facilitate a change in orientation from disease-based systems. There is a need for the development of public health systems that give preventative action as the highest priority and more appropriately target at-risk groups. This requires high levels of intersectorial cooperation and collaboration right from government through to local services. Nishtar *et al.* (2006) described the intersectorial cooperation in Pakistan where a partnership model involving government, non-government organisations and the WHO has guided the development of a national action plan on chronic disease. While outcomes of the partnership are yet to be realised, the strategy has aimed to obtain maximum benefit using the country's limited resources. Their approach has seen a horizontal integration of existing programmes to reorient health systems to include chronic illness, and arguably serves what previously was seen as two distinct populations within the country (those with chronic disease and those with communicable and acute disease).

Integrated approaches to chronic illness also reveal a need for greater investment in research that facilitates the transfer of scientific knowledge into practice. International priorities for research have been identified to include the determination of the best mix and organisation of strategies for chronic illness prevention, the continued efforts to develop cost-effective strategies for managing chronic illnesses and the impact of globalisation on risk and prevalence. Srinivasan and colleagues (2003), for example, discuss the need for interdisciplinary research related to the factors in the built environment that influence health and incorporate understanding, translating the outcomes of such work into practical policy and community actions to improve public health. Additionally, research needs to develop knowledge about the political aspects of health policy development and identify strategies to facilitate the earlier uptake of scientific knowledge about health promotion and prevention at all levels of government across the globe. There needs to be continued management of surveillance systems and sharing of data to support information sharing and trend analysis.

A further challenge for researchers involves bridging the gap between the current knowledge interests of developed and developing countries in understanding chronic illnesses and how the knowledge gained in one context might be applied to assist people in different contexts. Increased international research collaboration in addition to the existing global epidemiological studies is needed, particularly in addressing areas where issues are associated with the social determinants of health. International collaboration among low-, middle- and high-income countries could assist in the transference of knowledge and needs to address the current trend of unidirectional flow of knowledge.

Conclusion

There is now a greater acknowledgement and acceptance that there is a global epidemic of chronic illness that needs urgent broad-based action. While biomedical science remains important in understanding chronic illness, there has been a rapid shift in recognition of social and economic factors being instrumental in the increasing prevalence of chronic illnesses. The myth of chronic illness as linked to affluent lifestyles in developed countries has been debunked, and the burden of chronic illness is significantly greater in low- and middle-income countries.

Accompanying the recognition of the social determinants of health is a broader acceptance of the need to understand illness experiences from the perspectives of those who live with illness. Solutions to living with illness need to incorporate the expertise of people who have intimate knowledge of their illness experience. There is considerable knowledge now about the transitions people experience in the illness and the importance of relationships in managing those transitions. These relationships include health personnel who are increasingly challenged to work in partnership with people with chronic illness, rather than imposing their preferred approaches to care.

There are numerous challenges to developing effective strategies to reduce the burden of chronic illness for both individuals and their communities, as well as in creating systems of care to support those affected. Self-management is one of a number of strategies promoted to empower people to be in control of their care. However, there are risks in relying on this model alone; it potentially could act as a mechanism for the transference of responsibility from the state to individuals.

While there is vast research and associated knowledge creation across the globe related to chronic illness, there is minimal exploration of how the knowledge could be transferred and benefit nations of different socio-economic status. There are considerable opportunities for interdisciplinary and international collaboration to facilitate knowledge and resource sharing. These exchanges need to increase the flow of knowledge from less developed nations, rather than the most commonly occurring flow from developed nations to the rest of the world.

References

Allen, M. (2007) *Key Note Address: Students as Audiences: Learning from Media Studies/ Learning Through Media.* UB Flexible: Facing the Future: University of Ballarat Learning and Teaching Conference, July 2007, Ballarat.

Allsop, J., Jones, K., Baggott, R. (2004) Health consumer groups in the UK: a new social movement? *Sociology of Health and Illness* **26**(6): 737–756.

Beckmann, K., Strassnick, K., Abell, L., Hermann, J., Oakley, B. (2007) Is chronic disease self-management program beneficial to people affected by cancer? *Australian Journal of Primary Health* **13**(1): 36–44.

Charmaz, K. (2000) Experiencing chronic illness. In: Albrecht, G.L., Fitzpatrick, R., Scrimshaw, S.C. (eds) *The Handbook of Social Studies in Health and Medicine*. Sage Publications: London.

Clapton, J., Kendall, E. (2002) Autonomy and participation in rehabilitation: time for a new paradigm? *Disability and Rehabilitation* **24**(18): 987–991.

Dowrick, C. (2006) The chronic disease strategy for Australia. *Medical Journal of Australia* **185**(2): 61–62.

Doyal, L., Pennell, I. (1979) *The Political Economy of Health*. Pluto Press: London.

Fox, J. (2005) The role of the expert patient in the management of chronic illness. *British Journal of Nursing* **14**(1): 25–28.

Gerber, A., Hentzelt, F., Lauterbach, K.W. (2007) Can evidence-based medicine implicitly rely on current concepts of disease or does it have to develop its own definition? *Journal of Medical Ethics* **33**: 394–399.

Gifford, A.L., Laurent, D.D., Gonsales, V.M., Chesney, M.A., Lorig, K.R. (1998) Pilot randomized trial of education to improve self management skills of men with symptomatic HIV/AIDS. *Journal of AIDS* **18**(2): 136–144.

Hardy, M. (2002) The story of my illness: personal accounts of illness on the Internet. *Health (London)* **6**(1): 31–46.

Hofman, K., Ryce, A., Prudhomme, W., Kotzin, S. (2006) Reporting of non-communicable disease research in low- and middle-income countries: a pilot bibliometric analysis. *Journal of the Medical Library Association* **94**(4): 415–420.

Hofmann, B. (2002) On the triad disease, illness and sickness. *Journal of Medicine and Philosophy* **27**(6): 651–673.

Homer, J., Hirsch, G., Milstein, B. (2007) Chronic illness in a complex health economy: the perils and promises of downstream and upstream reforms. *System Dynamics Review* **23**(2–3): 313–343.

Horton, R. (2005) The neglected epidemic of chronic disease. *The Lancet* **366**(9496): 1514.

Irwin, A., Valentine, N., Brown, C. *et al.* (2006) The commission on social determinants of health: tackling the social roots of inequities. *PLoS Medicine* **3**(6): e106.

Judson, L. (2004) Global childhood chronic illness. *Nursing Administration Quarterly* **28**(1): 60–66.

Kelly, M.P., Field, D. (1996) Medical sociology, chronic illness and the body. *Sociology of Health and Illness* **18**(2): 241–257.

Kendall, E., Rogers, A. (2007) Extinguishing the social?: state sponsored self-care policy and the chronic disease self-management program. *Disability and Society* **22**(2): 129–143.

Kralik, D. (2002) The quest for ordinariness: transition experienced by midlife women living with chronic illness. *Journal of Advanced Nursing* **39**(2): 146–154.

Kralik, D., Visentin, K., van Loon, A. (2006) Transition: a literature review. *Journal of Advanced Nursing* **55**(3): 320–329.

Larsen, P.D. (2006) Chronicity. In: Lubkin, I.M., Larsen, P.D. (eds) *Chronic Illness: Impact and Interventions*, 3rd edition. Jones & Bartlett: Boston.

Le Galès-Camus, C. (2005) Fighting chronic disease. *Bulletin of the World Health Organization* **83**(6): 407–408.

Livneh, H. (2001) Psychosocial adaptation to chronic illness and disability: a conceptual framework. *Rehabilitation Counseling Bulletin* **44**(3): 151–160.

Livneh, H., Antonak, R.F. (2005) Psychosocial adaptation to chronic illness and disability: a primer for counselors. *Journal of Counseling and Development* **83**: 12–20.

Lorig, K.R., Holman, H.R. (2003) Self-management education: history, definition, outcomes, and mechanisms. *Annals of Behavioral Medicine* **26**(1): 1–7.

Lorig, K., Sobel, D., Stewart, A. *et al.* (1999) Evidence suggesting that a chronic disease self-management program can improve health status while reducing hospitalization: a randomized trial. *Medical Care* **37**: 5–14.

Lubkin, I.M., Larsen, P.D. (eds) (2006) *Chronic Illness: Impact and Interventions*, 3rd edition. Jones & Bartlett: Boston.

Marmot, M. (2005) Social determinants of health inequalities. *The Lancet* **365**: 1099–1104.

Mathers, C.D., Vos, E.T., Stevenson, C.E., Begg, S.J. (2001) The burden of disease and injury in Australia. *Bulletin of the World Health Organization* **79**(11): 1076–1084.

McGrath, P., Henderson, D., Holewa, H. (2006) Patient-centred care: qualitative findings on health professionals' understandings of ethics in acute medicine. *Bioethical Inquiry* **3**: 149–160.

Mengshoel, A.M., Heggen, K.M. (2004) Recovery from fibromyalgia – previous patients' own experiences. *Disability and Rehabilitation* **26**(1): 46–53.

Miller, J.F. (2000) *Coping with Chronic Illness: Overcoming Powerlessness*. F.A. Davis Company: Philadelphia, PA.

Nishtar, S., Bille, K.M., Ahmed, A., *et al.* (2006) Process, rationale, and interventions of Pakistan's national action plan on chronic diseases. *Preventing Chronic Disease: Public Health Research, Practice and Policy* (serial online) **3**(1), available from http://www.cdc.gov/pcd/issues/2006/jan/05_0066.htm (accessed 15 December 2007).

O'Halloran, J., Britt, H., Valenti, L., Harrison, C., Pan, Y., Knox, S. (2003) *Older Patients Attending General Practice in Australia 2000–2002*, General Practice Series, Vol. 12, AIHW Cat. No. GEP 12. Australian Institute of Health and Welfare: Canberra.

Penney, W. (2005) *A Critical ethnographic study of older people participating in their health care in acute hospital environments*. Unpublished PhD Thesis, University of Ballarat.

Penney, W., Wellard, S. (2007) Hearing what older consumers say about participation in their care. *International Journal of Nursing Practice* **13**: 61–68.

Prentice, A.M. (2006) The emerging epidemic of obesity in developing countries. *International Journal of Epidemiology* **35**: 93–99.

Price, B. (1996) Illness careers: the chrome illness experience. *Journal of Advanced Nursing* **24**(2): 275–279.

Rasmussen, B., O'Connell, B., Dunning, P., Cox, H. (2007) Young women with type 1 diabetes' management of turning points and transitions. *Qualitative Health Research* **17**: 300–310.

Srinivasan, S., O'Fallon, L.R., Dearry, A. (2003) Creating healthy communities, healthy homes, healthy people: initiating a research agenda on the built environment and public health. *American Journal of Public Health* **93**(9): 1446–1450.

Strong, K., Mathers, C., Epping-Jordan, J. (2006) Preventing chronic disease: a priority for global health. *International Journal of Epidemiology* **35**(2): 492–494.

Strong, K., Mathers, C., Leeder, S., Beaglehole, R. (2005) Preventing chronic diseases: how many lives can we save? *The Lancet* **366**: 1578–1582.

Taylor, B. (2005) Health, wellness, illness, healing and holism and nursing. In: Rogers-Clark, C., McCarthy, A., Martin-McDonald, K. (eds) *Living with Illness: Psychosocial Challenges for Nursing*. Elsevier: Sydney.

Taylor, D., Bury, M. (2007) Chronic illness, patient experts and care transition. *Sociology of Health and Illness* **29**(1): 27–45.

Thorne, S.E. (2006) Patient–provider communication in chronic illness: a health promotion opportunity. *Family and Community Health* **29**(1S): 4s–11s.

Thorne, S.E., Paterson, B.L. (2000) Two decades of insider research: what we know and don't know about chronic illness experience. *Annual Review of Nursing Research* **18**: 3–25.

Tinetti, M.E., Fried, T. (2004) The end of the disease era. *American Journal of Medicine* **116**: 179–185.

Walker, C. (2007) Chronic illness and consumer inequality: the impact of health costs on people with chronic illnesses in rural and regional Victoria. *Australian Health Review* **31**(2): 203–210.

Weeramanthri, T., Hendy, S., Connors, C. *et al.* (2003) The Northern Territory preventable chronic disease strategy – promoting an integrated and life course approach to chronic disease in Australia. *Australian Health Review* **26**(3): 31–42.

Wellard, S.J. (1998) Constructions of chronic illness. *International Journal of Nursing Studies* **35**: 49–55.

Wellard, S.J., Beddoes, L. (2005) Constructions of chronic illness. In: Rogers-Clark, C., Martin-McDonald, K., McCathy, A. (eds) *Living with Illness: Psychosocial Challenges. A Text for Nurses and Other Caring Professionals*. Elsevier Churchill Livingstone: Sydney.

Wellard, S.J., Cox, H., Bhujoharry, C. (2007) Issues in the provision of nursing care to people undergoing cardiac surgery who also have type 2 diabetes. *International Journal of Nursing Practice* **13**: 222–228.

Wellard, S.J., Lillibridge, J., Beanland, C.J., Lewis, M. (2003) Consumer participation in acute care settings: an Australian experience. *International Journal of Nursing Practice* **9**: 255–260.

Werner, A., Widding Isaksen, L., Malterud, K. (2004) 'I am not the kind of woman who complains of everything': illness stories on self and shame in women with chronic pain. *Social Science and Medicine* **59**(5): 1035–1045.

Wikman, A., Marklund, S., Alexanderson, K. (2005) Illness, disease, and sickness absence: an empirical test of differences between concepts of ill health. *Journal of Epidemiology and Community Health* **59**(6): 450–454.

Wilde, M.H. (2003) Embodied knowledge in chronic illness and injury. *Nursing Inquiry* **10**(3): 170–176.

Wilkinson, R., Marmot, M. (2003) *The Solid Facts*. World Health Organization: Copenhagen.

Woolf, S.H., Chan, E.C.Y., Harris, R. *et al.* (2005) Promoting informed consent: transforming health care to dispense knowledge for decision making. *Annals of Internal Medicine* **143**: 293–300.

World Health Organization (WHO) (2005) *Preventing Chronic Disease: A Vital Investment: WHO Global Report*. WHO: Geneva. http://www.who.int/chp/chronic_disease_report/en/ (accessed September 2007).

Yach, D., Hawkes, C., Gould, C.L., Hofman, K.J. (2004) The global burden of chronic diseases: overcoming impediments to prevention and control. *Journal of the American Medical Association* **291**(21): 2616–2622.

2. *Transitional Processes and Chronic Illness*

Debbie Kralik and Antonia van Loon

Introduction

People can experience the impact of chronic or long-term illness to be life changing. Adapting and adjusting to life with chronic illness involves learning to live with unwanted change. Illness can be erratic and unpredictable, requiring constant life adjustments. A chronic illness can bring many overt and subtle changes into a person's life, such as changes to employment and income, identity and relationships, parenting, life priorities and changes to physical, mental, emotional, social and spiritual well-being. People with chronic illness can experience these changes as losses, including loss of control, independence, familiar lifestyle, meaning, purpose and hope. In addition, people face the possible relinquishing of their dreams and aspirations for the future as they face the fear of continuing and ongoing losses. Changing roles in family, work and social situations resulting from a person's illness also can create adjustment issues for everyone relating to the ill person in an ongoing relationship.

Health professionals often have to work with people who are learning to adapt to the significant changes of living with chronic illness. Some health professionals focus on problematising and pathologising health and illness. People learning to live with illness in their life context may view this approach as fragmented and unsatisfactory. When health professionals understand the transition process and the ways they can help people to incorporate the consequences of chronic illness into their lives, they will see that they are able to make a substantial contribution to enable people to recognise their needs, make informed choices, effectively self-care and develop their personal capacity to incorporate the future change that accompanies many chronic conditions.

Transitional life events such as separation, divorce, redundancy, family violence, chronic illness, disability and dying can cause disruption to one's sense of self. Even anticipated changes such as the birth of a child, retirement, relocation or marriage may produce disruption. These disruptive events create an end to a person's familiar ways of living and require the individual to find new ways to live and be in the world. Understanding transition involves exploring the person's responses to a passage of circumstances and events that demand life adjustment. The process of living involves the need for transition, requiring humans to adjust and modify their responses, behaviours and attitudes to ever-changing life situations. Most of this modification goes on unnoticed. However, the changes associated with the presence of altered health and the permanence of having a chronic illness may cause significant disruption to the person's sense of self. It is the transition through the changes associated with learning to live with chronic illness that is the focus of this chapter.

This chapter builds upon previous and ongoing research with people experiencing disruptions such as chronic illness and community-based health professionals. The aim of this research programme has been to develop an understanding of the concept of transition and how it can inform health practice. We begin by exploring how the concept of transition has been reported in the literature and applied in research and practice settings. We then present a framework to understand the transition that has emerged from our own research programme in the community health context, aiming to assist health professionals to consider how they may facilitate personal transition when working with people.

The search

A preliminary search using transition as a keyword retrieved an enormous volume of work, making it clear that the search needed to be radically narrowed. The inclusion criteria for articles were as follows:

- Articles were dated between 1994 and 2008.
- Transition was a central concept.
- The focus was on chronic illness.

Meleis and Trangenstein (1994) had previously reviewed transition literature published prior to 1994, so our intention was to build on this work and focus on literature published after that date. Databases (MEDLINE, CINAHL, Sociofile, Psychlit) were searched using *transition* and a query string of *social*, *life events*, *illness*, *crisis*, *identity* and *self*. The focus of transition in articles in MEDLINE was molecular or biological in nature, so these articles were excluded. There was some overlap within the searches, but additional articles were identified once combinations were included. Sociofile and Psychlit retrieved a number of articles that focused on identity and social life. We manually searched the reference lists of the reviewed articles for additional relevant sources. To further extend the theoretical understanding of transition, the terms *continuity*, *identity*, *personhood*, *self*, *agency* and *disruption* were added to the search. Full transcripts of relevant articles ($n = 47$) were located.

A total of 22 articles were excluded from the final review. Four articles focused on transition as life or developmental stages, so these were excluded (Mann *et al.* 1999; Sawyer 1999; Draper 2003; Nelson 2003). The authors of a further 18 articles used the word *transition* without describing the concept (Montenko & Greenberg 1995; White 1995; Brudenell 1996; Gwilliam & Bailey 2001; Brouwer-Dudokdewit *et al.* 2002; Vaartio *et al.* 2003; White 2003; Forss *et al.* 2004); therefore these articles had limited use for this chapter and were excluded.

Defining transition

The word *transition* is derived from the Latin word *transitio* that means going across – passage over time, stage, subject or one place to another – that is, to change (Lexico 2005). Transition has been used in diverse ways across the academic literature of disciplines as varied as musicology, history, metallurgy, geography, anthropology, science and health, with discussions ranging from change at the molecular level to personal and developmental changes, to global countries in transition. Authors have frequently used the word transition to describe a process of change in life's developmental stages, the movement from one situation to another or alterations in health and social circumstances.

Transition is not an event, but rather the 'inner reorientation and self-redefinition' that people go through to incorporate change into their life (Bridges 2004, p. xii). Definitions of transition alter depending on the disciplinary focus, but most state that transition involves a passage of change. A common definition of *transition* cited in health disciplines is

> *A passage from one life phase, condition, or status to another . . . transition refers to both the process and the outcome of complex person–environment interactions. It may involve more than one person and is embedded in the context and the situation. Defining characteristics of transition include process, disconnectedness perception and patterns and response.*
>
> *(Chick & Meleis 1986, pp. 239–240)*

The concept of transition has evolved in the social science and health disciplines during the past three decades. Interestingly, nurses have made significant contributions to recent understandings of the transition process as it relates to life and health (Chick & Meleis 1986; Cantanzaro 1990; Loveys 1990; Meleis & Trangenstein 1994; Schumacher & Meleis 1994; Meleis *et al.* 2000; Kralik 2002; van Loon & Kralik 2005a, 2005b; Kralik *et al.* 2006a, 2006b, 2006c).

An emerging understanding of transition

Transition theory has a long history within other disciplines, especially anthropology. Van Gennep's (1960) theory proposed that people move through life's stages in three distinct phases. First, pre-liminal rites (rites of separation) are characterised by removal of the individual from their 'normal' social life, which may occur through the use of customs and taboos. Secondly the liminal rites (rites of transition) refer to customs and rituals of the individual when they are in a liminal state, perhaps feeling confused and alienated, in a state of 'limbo' or as Draper (2003, p. 63) prefers, 'in no man's land'. Finally, the post liminal rites (rites of incorporation) occur where the individuals are brought back into society and take up their new status (re-incorporation). Van Gennep's three-phase approach to transition continues to influence current thinking about transition published in the social and health literature. For example, three phases to transition have also been proposed by Bridges (2004, p. 17), where 'first there is an ending, then a beginning, and an important empty or fallow time in between'.

The work of Van Gennep (1960) was further developed by Turner (1969) and then Sheehy (1977) who proposed that 'rites of passage' throughout the stages of human life are marked by socio-cultural rituals. Martin-McDonald and Biernoff (2002, p. 347) suggest that 'rites of passage occur when there is a transition in cultural expectations, social roles, and status and/or condition or position, interpersonal relations, and developmental or situational changes to being in the world'. Bridges (2004) proposes that traditional societies facilitate transition by having rituals that assist people in the transition process by preparing them to let go of an outlived life phase and continue their sense of self, as they move through to the next phase of life.

These theorists offer frameworks in which the transition process can be studied. The common elements to transition theories are

1. a disconnection from previous social connections and supports;
2. an absence of familiar reference points (objects or persons);
3. the appearance of new needs and/or the inability to meet old needs in accustomed ways; and
4. the incongruence between a former set of roles, expectations and identity markers and those that prevail within the new situation.

Additionally, what these theories have in common is that a transition is a linear trajectory that involves a distinct start and finishing point. Other authors suggest that transition experiences are neither linear nor time bound (Glacken *et al.* 2001), but may be a cyclical process that revolves as it is enacted, to move through disruptive life changes (Kralik 2002).

Transition is the movement people make through a disruptive life event so that they can continue to live with a coherent and continuing sense of self (Kralik *et al.* 2006a, 2006b, 2006c). Transition is the reorientation and redefinition that people go through in order to incorporate changed circumstances into their lives (Bridges 2004). Transition occurs when a person's current reality is disrupted causing a forced or chosen change that results in the need to construct a new reality (Selder 1989). Transition can only occur if the person is aware of the changes that are taking place (Chick & Meleis 1986). This point is critical because often people in the midst of a disruptive life event may not be able to identify precisely what has/is changed/changing. They know their life is impacted and they may even be uncomfortable knowing that things are different, but they cannot say why this is causing so much disquiet and disruption. We posit that this is why some people do not engage in transition and feel overwhelmed by what they are experiencing. Health professionals often focus on the need for change through health promotion and patient education but they rarely focus on how people can be assisted to achieve transition where modifications are actually incorporated into a new way of living and being in the world.

A concept analysis of transition was published by Meleis *et al.* (2000) that provided, both, a perspective and a framework for defining the concept of transition such as developmental, health, socio-cultural, situational, relational, critical events and organisational changes. It was proposed that people may undergo more than one transition at any given time and it is important for the person to be aware of the changes taking place and to engage with them. According to this framework, a possible indicator that transition is occurring is that the persons feel connected to, and are interacting with, their situation, confronting the issues and/or people around them to gain an understanding of how to live and be in their altered world. The persons feel located or situated, so they can reflect and interact, and develop increasing confidence in their capacity to cope and live with the adjustments they must make. They master new skills and new ways of living while developing a more flexible and modified sense of identity in the midst of these changes (Meleis *et al.* 2000).

Meleis *et al.* (2000) suggest that awareness of change is followed by immersion in the process that facilitates transition and engaging in activities such as seeking information or support, identifying new ways of living and being, modifying former activities and making sense of the circumstances. Therefore a person's level of awareness will influence his or her level of engagement, with lack of awareness signifying that an individual may not be ready for transition (Meleis *et al.* 2000).

Both Bridges (2004) and Selder (1989) highlight the importance of a person's need to acknowledge that a prior way of living/being has ended or that a current reality is under threat and that change needs to occur before the transition process can begin. Once this acknowledgment occurs, a person can begin to make sense of what is happening and reorganise a new way to live, respond and be in the world. The process of surfacing awareness involves noticing what has changed and how things are different (Meleis *et al.* 2000; Kralik 2002). Dimensions of difference that can be explored include the nature of the change, how long the change will occur, what possible trajectory the change may follow, the perceived importance and severity of the change and the personal, familial and societal influences impacting on the changes (Meleis *et al.* 2000). Kralik (2002) proposes that people with chronic illness feel different from others and may be perceived by others as being different. They view their world in an altered way as a result of the movement that occurs during transition.

Describing transition

Transition is described as a passage or movement that incorporates a time of inner reorientation and/or transformation (Powell-Cope 1995; Shaul 1997;

Neil & Barrell 1998; Fraser 1999; Glacken *et al.* 2001; Elmberger *et al.* 2002; Hilton 2002; Kralik 2002; Arman & Rehnsfeldt 2003; Skarsater *et al.* 2003). The experience of transition has also been described as a process in response to disruptions in close relationships and daily living (Powell-Cope 1995; Arman & Rehnsfeldt 2003). It includes themes involving a loss of self or shifts in self-identity as a result of the uncertainty and turmoil that follow a crisis event or disruption (Neil & Barrell 1998; Glacken *et al.* 2001; Elmberger *et al.* 2002; Hilton 2002; Kralik 2002; Martin-McDonald & Biernoff 2002). These researchers found that people sought to recover control following the disruptive event and a reconstruction of self-identity was observed as the regaining of a sense of control or mastery.

To assist people to move towards a sense of mastery involves the acquisition of relevant information (Fraser 1999; Hilton 2002) and social support systems (Powell-Cope 1995; Rossen 1998; Martin-McDonald & Biernoff 2002). Other authors focused on transition as the adjustment and response to change that occurs during the course of progressive chronic illness, such as commencing dialysis, commencing insulin (Martin-McDonald & Biernoff 2002; Kralik *et al.* 2003) or learning to live with a permanent indwelling urinary catheter (Kralik *et al.* 2007). It is evident in this body of literature that transition is not simply change. Rather, it includes the sense-making process that people go through to incorporate the change or disruption into their lives (van Loon & Kralik 2007).

The transitional process has been described as involving transformation or alteration, whether it is incorporation, integration or adaptation to a change event. Transition has also been described as involving a process of inner reorientation as the person learns to adapt and incorporate the new circumstances into his or her life.

Transition and identity

A striking finding by a number of authors is the challenge to self-identity that occurs during the transition process. It is proposed that a difficult part of the transition with chronic illness is the adjustment to the identity one held before the onset of chronic illness (Kralik 2002; Bridges 2004). The transition process involves restructuring the way one defines oneself and the ways in which one interacts with the world (Kralik *et al.* 2007). Transition is linked to the notion of self and identity and how it is impacted upon by disruption (Boeije *et al.* 2002; Kralik 2002; Young *et al.* 2002). Self-identity is threatened during disruption and there is a need for reconstruction of identity based on altered roles and responsibilities (Luborsky 1994; Boeije *et al.* 2002; Young *et al.* 2002). Other authors exploring life transitions also focus on the process of shifts in identity and redefining of self (Bailey 1999; Banister 1999; Miller 2000). The importance of maintaining relationships and connections is identified as an integral part of successful transition (Meleis *et al.* 2000; Kralik *et al.* 2003; Bridges 2004). Researchers suggest that for transition to occur, people require social support systems (Glacken *et al.* 2002), maintaining or developing strong connections with others (Arman & Rehnsfeldt 2003) and learning ways to adapt to change through a heightened awareness of self (Shaul 1997; Fraser 1999; Hilton 2002; Kralik 2002; Martin-McDonald & Biernoff 2002; Kralik *et al.* 2003, 2007).

The process involved in transition may include increased suffering in the early stages but this suffering reduces over time as the person undertakes sense-making activities to understand the impacts of his or her changing circumstances and realigns his or her sense of self. The suffering invoked by forced change may be the driving motivation for transformation and, consequently, transition. For example, older women who have survived a stroke experience a process of transformation that results in a reconstruction of the sense of self (Hilton 2002). Women seek new roles, identify new coping strategies and reconcile with the limitations that the stroke imposes. Arman and Rehnsfeldt (2003) add that illness experiences can change one's notion of self, which Elmberger *et al.* (2002) claim may be 'processed' to 'master' the changing sense of identity and family relations imposed by the illness trajectory. Disruptive events, however, may increase suffering when the altered sense of self is difficult to reconcile to, but this may be ameliorated during the reclaiming or reorientating process that occurs during transition (Kralik 2002; Bridges 2004; van Loon & Kralik 2005a, 2005b).

Arman and Rehnsfeldt (2003) provide examples of studies where women were classified as 'stuck' and unable to transition because they were not able to adapt and integrate cancer into their lives. Other authors assume that all people transition successfully through an illness experience because they provide little or no discussion around people who have not experienced transition (Hilton 2002; Skarsater *et al.* 2003).

There were some studies where participants identified transition as an important part of healing and recovery (Glacken *et al.* 2001; Kralik 2002). Participants describe the process of reconstructing and incorporating change as essential to transition, whether it is in the context of relationships, roles or strategies for coping (Hilton 2002; Skarsater *et al.* 2003). van Loon and Kralik's (2005a, 2005b, 2007) analysis of interviews with women challenged by homelessness, chronic illness and addiction revealed that transition can involve reworking a complex interplay of learned maladaptive activities. These women had to work out what aspects of their old self they could hold on to, and what they had to relinquish to move forward with life. As homeless women, they were dislocated and disconnected from family relationships, with no sense of predictability and permanence in roles, status, location or situation. Their security came from numbing away their suffering using addictive substances and behaviours. Their sense of self-identity was largely shaped by guilt, shame, fear and anger. They had to incorporate massive changes brought on by their choice to enter recovery programmes. This required each woman to recognise what was changing, acknowledge their discomfort, and seek new ways to manage that struggle within themselves. They needed to be prepared to live with the sense of dislocation, confusion and uncertainty that came with reorienting their life towards a drug- or alcohol- and gambling-free future. When you do not like or esteem the self that you face each day, it is very confronting and anxiety-provoking to do this activity, so great support needs to be provided at this point of care. van Loon and Kralik (2005a, 2005b, 2007) note that these women found within themselves and their support group ways to reorient their sense of self, reconnect with others, revise their values and reclaim themselves. The net result was an improved capacity to negotiate changes and transition to a more preferred future that included physical, psychological and spiritual healing, and reconciliation with their children and families over time.

Transition and transformative learning

Over time, people accumulate an increasing reservoir of experience that becomes a resource for learning. Learning to live with chronic illness can be hard work as people renegotiate meaning in many aspects of their lives, grieve their losses and attend to the practicalities of treatments/interventions and appointments. People do attach meaning to the learning they gain from experiences, even if they were adverse and difficult. It enables some people to embrace their struggle and suffering and say that they have gained a depth of wisdom and understanding about life and what is valuable, which is impossible to garner in other ways (van Loon & Kralik 2006).

This transformative learning is a part of the transition process. Transformative learning is considered to be the kind of learning people undertake when making meaning of their lives (Cranton 1996). Mezirow (2000) posits that all learning is change but not all change is transformation because people may not follow transformational processes. Meaning is constructed from acquired knowledge. He proposes that people move through phases when they experience transformation learning. Those steps are as follows:

- Experiencing a disorienting dilemma
- Self-examination
- Critical assessment of assumptions
- Recognising that others have gone through a similar process
- Exploring options
- Formulating a plan of action
- Reintegration

Transformative learning is triggered by a challenge. After identifying the problem or challenge, people enter a phase where they reflect critically. During the thinking phase, people may find that they can no longer keep their old ways of thinking and being, and are compelled to change. There is also a phase where people plan and take action to integrate change into their lives. It is evident through this brief description that there are links between transition and transformative learning theories. There appears to be an element of critical thinking to transformative learning. When using critical thinking the person makes a decision or solves a problem in a reflective way. We have found that the simple approach of 'look, think and act' promotes the thinking that facilitates the transformative action that leads to transition. This approach is described later in this chapter.

It is assumed that transformative learning requires a teacher to foster the process and play a key role; however, we know that transition occurs often by a person's own internal dialogue and thinking. We posit that the health professional can facilitate the internal dialogue that facilitates transformative learning by establishing a relational environment that facilitates this thinking and by providing tools to assist critical reflection and self-understanding. The goal of this transformative learning is to share the activities and experience of meaning-making. All participants in the process should demonstrate a willingness to learn and support each other to make changes (Torosyan 2007). We contend that these principles facilitate transition effectively when they are used in self-help and support groups. We believe that health professionals will be better equipped to assist people with the adaptation and adjustment required for transition if they have some understanding of the process and some tools to progress people through the change process. Few processes to facilitate transition have been identified in the health literature; yet we know that translating knowledge into practice that can affect client outcomes requires applied and practical processes.

Transitional processes

There is a lack of consensus among researchers as to whether the dynamic transition process has a definite beginning and an end, is linear or cyclical and how it is that health care practitioners can best help people to 'move on'. Research reports in which Van Gennep's rites of passage theory are used as a theoretical frame (Luborsky 1994; Froggatt 1997; Martin-McDonald & Biernoff 2002) tend to assume that transition is linear and uni-directional, even suggesting that the three phases are somehow distinct and readily separated for examination. Likewise, other authors propose that transition has a beginning and an end (Fraser 1999; Elmberger *et al.* 2002; Bridges 2004). However, Kralik (2002) suggests that transition is cyclical because change is a constant force in human life. For example, Elmberger *et al.* (2002) describe how men with cancer commence the health–illness transition at diagnosis and how the transitional period lasts for several years, experienced in a spiral movement. Likewise Paterson (2001, 2003), after undertaking a meta-synthesis of 292 qualitative research studies, describes a 'shifting perspectives' model of chronic illness that challenges the notion of a linear trajectory in transition. She proposes that living with a chronic illness is an ongoing transformational process involving movement in many directions. Glacken *et al.* (2001) suggest that the transitional process is unique, neither time bound nor linear in nature, and the duration and outcomes are different for each individual.

There is frequent reference to the course of change associated with breast cancer as a type of 'transition', 'transformation', 'transcendence' encompassing a search for 'meaning' as one travels a path that aims to regain 'integrity', 'balance' and 'wholeness' within the person. Arman and Rehnsfeldt (2003) reveal that women can be in different phases of a transitional process and move between them simultaneously. Powell-Cope (1995, p. 54) states that the transition process is not linear but recurring, so that at any given time new losses require ongoing readjustments; thus, transition continues throughout life. It has also been proposed that while many life transitions have a distinct beginning and end, transition for people with chronic illness may be ongoing, as one's health and well-being fluctuates (Shaul 1997).

A limitation of the transition and chronic illness research reported is its short-term focus. The passage of time is an essential element in transition and as such, longitudinal studies are required that explore experiences that lead to transition (Powell-Cope 1995; Shaul 1997; Rossen 1998; Fraser 1999; Hilton 2002; Kralik 2002; Martin-McDonald & Biernoff 2002; Kralik *et al.* 2003). Fraser (1999) used multiple interviews with participants over time to describe transition. Kralik (2002) used email and letter-writing correspondence as a longitudinal data-generation strategy in her study with women with chronic illness, to discover that women move through a phase of 'extraordinariness' in which they are in turmoil and distress, but they may move back into a sense of ordinariness as changes are amalgamated. This is never a stepping process, rather it is a non-linear 'to and fro' movement, that recurs but steadily moves forward (Kralik 2002).

van Loon and Kralik's (2005a, 2005b, 2006, 2007) research with women recovering from addiction who were moving from supported accommodation to independent housing found that the women experienced transition as many movements forward and backward and sometimes even a slipping way back in an almost 'snakes and ladders' type walk through life. As new issues challenged them and ongoing changes had to be incorporated into a new way of living without alcohol and drugs, their movements were anything but linear in nature; yet, over time they were moving forward and transitioning from their past.

A transition framework for practice

It has been argued that the planning and implementation of health-care activities could be informed by the concept of transition (Shaul 1997). Glacken *et al.* (2001) suggested that a tool should be developed that assists health professionals to assess where the person is within the transition process, thus ensuring that appropriate strategies are implemented at the right times. Preliminary work on such a tool has commenced pertaining to survivors of child sexual abuse (van Loon & Kralik 2005a, 2005b). Using such tools may provide a framework to build capacity by planning strategies that assist sense-making activities, enabling the person to decide what can be kept from his or her past and what must be relinquished in order to move forward through the various stages of transition (van Loon & Kralik 2005a, 2005b).

During the past decade, we have undertaken more than 60 individual research projects where the findings have contributed like building blocks to a transition framework that could inform community health practice. Our research programme has involved researching with people challenged by disruptive events such as the onset of chronic illness. We have utilised a collaborative research approach, guided by primary health-care (PHC) principles and participatory action research (PAR) (Wadsworth 1991, 1998; Stringer 1999; Orlanda 2001; Reason & Bradbury 2001; Williamson & Prosser 2002).

In this programme of research, we have come to understand transition as a complex life process during which persons realign their sense of self-identity and redevelop self-agency in response to disruption (Kralik *et al.* 2006a, 2006b, 2006c). When undertaking the work of realigning one's sense of self-identity, it is helpful if the persons come to an understanding of what has changed in their life so that they can see how their current reality is shifting or has shifted (Kralik 2002). The persons examine the nature of the change and the possibility, or otherwise, of returning to their familiar life. They can investigate how long this change is likely to be present and if life is going to be permanently altered. The persons may need help to see the possibilities that may be opening up, since the change event has ended their former way of living and being in the world. This exploratory process allows health professionals or others working with people with chronic illness to highlight opportunities and diminish the threats posed by the change experience. Together, the person and the health professional can explore the significance and difficulty of the changes and the personal, familial, social and spiritual influences that are impacted by, or impacting on, the change.

The person acknowledges that a prior way of living/being has ended, or a current reality is under threat, and that change needs to occur for the transition process to begin (Selder 1989; Bridges 2004; van Loon & Kralik 2005a, 2005b, 2007). Once acknowledged, the person can feel and grieve his or her losses. This is often a time of great emotional turmoil, stress, confusion and suffering where even simple tasks may be experienced as overwhelming (van Loon & Kralik 2005a, 2005b, 2006, 2007).

Transition takes time as people disengage with what was known and familiar and find a new way to locate themselves in an altered world. The health professional can facilitate this process by providing a safe space to listen to people's stories, so that they can hear their own words and explore new perspectives on those stories. In the dialogue, the persons will find the values that they hold and perspectives of themselves that they wish to reclaim and those they need/want to discard surfacing. This facilitates the required sense-making that enables the person to effect change.

Without such examination of the change events, the person's understanding of what shifting is may be limited (Telford *et al.* 2006). People need the opportunity to examine their perceptions and see how they motivate and sustain their actions to change over time. There may not be a discrete start or end point in the transition process because change is a part of life, but change that impacts the person's sense of self is the issue of concern to health professionals. Signs that transition is occurring include reconnection to, and interaction with, other people (Meleis *et al.* 2000). The person feels connected and has a sense of belonging (van Loon & Kralik 2007). As the person develops new life skills, his or her coping strategies improve and he or she develops a more flexible perspective about who he or she perceives himself or herself to be in this new situation. It is this adaptive capacity in a world of challenge that helps resilience and personal capacity to grow (Young-Eisendrath 1996).

Transition involves backward and forward movement over time, but to facilitate understanding we have simplified transition into four phases. This framework of transition has been influenced by earlier work of theorists and builds on their understandings (Van Gennep 1960; Meleis & Trangenstein 1994; Becker 1997; McAdams *et al.* 2001; Bridges 2004). The focus has been on understanding the restorative processes that people experience when they adapt to change forced by an adverse situation so that people again experience a sense of becoming ordinary. The phases of transition identified in our research are (see Figure 2.1)

- the familiar life;
- the change event/disrupting experience that causes an ending;
- the limbo phase where the person is neither in his or her familiar former life nor has he or she incorporated the changes required to move into a new way of living; and finally
- the phase of becoming ordinary where changes are integrated and the person has located a sense of self with which he or she is able to live and function with a sense of continuous self (van Loon & Kralik 2005a, 2005b, 2006, 2007).

Familiar life

Before the change event occurs, people experience their life as something familiar. They have predictable lives, roles, status and identity. There is a sense of certainty and security in everyday experiences and relationships. The ordinary is captured in the routines and repetitions of daily living. The person knows what to expect and even if that is not desirable it is known. In this familiar life the person knows his or her social roles, cultural norms and the labels and social expectations attached to those positions. This knowledge creates a sense of familiar order.

The change event that produces an ending

People view the change event as an ending to their 'familiar' life. Life is full of endings. All people move through various developmental stages, employment, roles and relationships. Many endings are amalgamated without any sense of disruption. Some changes are anticipated with excitement and optimism; however, other endings cause trouble and interrupt one's sense of self. A medical diagnosis of a long-term illness or life-limiting disease may cause a person, and his or her significant others, profound disruption.

The change event causes interruption to the normal patterns of living and being in the world. For example, when illness intervenes in life old ways of living and responding no longer work and new ways to live have to be developed. The change may be desirable and exciting, or obligatory and terrifying, or anything in between. The disruption ends the known way of living and forces the person to modify connections or anchor points in the social world (van Loon & Kralik 2005a, 2005b, 2007).

FAMILIAR LIFE	ENDING	LIMBO	BECOMING ORDINARY

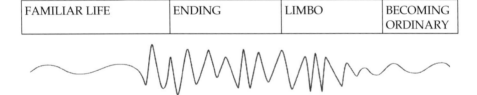

The graph represents movement occurring during each phase of the transition process. Disruption changes familiar life patterns and forces the person into a 'Limbo' period where they must make sense of the changes so they can relocate new ways to live and be in the world.

Living in familiar and predictable situations can be taken for granted.	The familiar way of living ends. The change event may be chosen or forced, but life is different.	The change becomes disorientating. It can be a time of suffering. Moving through this phase is facilitated by sense-making activities.	Changing patterns of being and doing are incorporated into new ways of living. Life is lived in a way that provides a sense of coherence.
In familiar life patterns people experience: • predictability • identity • roles • status • location • situation • security • relationships • connections • acquaintances • internalised socio-cultural norms • thoughts, feelings, attitudes within self • ordinary life	Following an ending people may experience: • disruption • difference • fractured identity • brokenness • overburden • displacement • separation • disconnection • uncertainty • hesitation • insecurity • ambiguity • vulnerability • inadequacy • violation • victimisation	During 'Limbo' people may experience: • confusion • turmoil • uncertainty • confrontation • alienation • isolation • loneliness • self-absorption • self-pity • incongruence • unanchored betrayal • powerlessness • loss and grief • insecurity • disenfranchised • extraordinariness • suffering	In becoming ordinary, people may experience: • realignment • reconstructing • revising • revaluing • reconnecting • reclaiming • refining • reconciling • relocation • renewal • coexisting • new beginnings • transformation • growth • progress • continuity • familiarity • resilience • healing • mastery • a return to ordinary life • feeling 'normal'

Figure 2.1 The four phases of transition (van Loon & Kralik 2005a, 2005b, 2006, 2007; Kralik *et al.* 2006a, 2006b, 2006c).

Limbo

People will move into a state that is neither in the past nor in the future. They may feel powerless and victimised, particularly if the changes are imposed. 'Limbo' is a time where people's sense of difference heightens and consequently they can feel isolated, alienated and alone. They may feel relegated to oblivion, where they are forced to disregard and forget who they were and not certain of who they will become with the imposed changes of chronic illness. One of the functions of 'Limbo' is to acknowledge what has changed and identify the accompanying losses and allow one's self to grieve those losses. People may feel overwhelmed by their loss and grief, which can intensify when they do the introspection and exploration of those losses with a health professional.

The task for health professionals working with people in 'Limbo' is to commence the sense-making process, to work out the new anchor points that enable one to locate oneself within the changing circumstances. Some people can live in this 'Limbo' state for years, being unable to move forward and/or backward with life and being stuck in this lonely hiatus, searching for a way by which they can recapture their sense of self (van Loon & Kralik 2005a, 2005b, 2007). If people spend too long in the self-absorbed state of 'Limbo', they can quickly move towards increasing self-pity and depression. If people do not take the time to recognise and reconcile their losses they may find that they are unable to move forwards because they are hampered by anger and resentment. The role of the health professional can be to facilitate sense-making activities within the therapeutic relationship.

The new beginning that leads to becoming ordinary

After people have made sense of their changing circumstances they can then incorporate the changes created by the alteration in their role, status, personhood or way of life. As they incorporate changes and develop a stronger sense of self they increase their resilience and build their capacity to overcome adversity. These successes build confidence, which in turn motivates the people to take increased personal responsibility in their life.

Success develops perseverance, ignites hope and increases the self-agency that enables the person to live independently with decreasing need for professional support. The newness of this way of life must be incorporated and the persons face significant choices that they must act on. Over time the persons will discover familiar landscape markers that reveal a new social landscape and their place within it which allows the continuity of identity.

Facilitating transition

Promoting the sense-making processes is the key to facilitating transition. 'Look, Think, Act' (explained subsequently) is a simple approach that assists people in working out what is happening in their lives. 'Look, Think, Act' focuses on changing, thinking and challenging routine behaviours so that people can antici-pate future behaviours and select their responses more carefully and act on their choices so that they may obtain different outcomes under similar circumstances.

This simple process facilitates the important life function of maintaining and nurturing a coherent sense of self-identity within changing and ambiguous life circumstances.

The 'look, think, act' process

Health professionals can facilitate transition using the 'look, think, act' process (Stringer 1996, 1999; Stringer & Genat 2004).

'*Look*' means find the issue, find out what is going on. Commence by allowing the person to tell his or her story in an uninterrupted and safe space so that he or she knows that he or she is being heard (van Loon & Kralik 2005a, 2005b, 2007). Instead of beginning a conversation with the person focusing on the disease, try asking, 'Tell me what concerns you most', 'Tell me what is most difficult for you at this time'. It will help if the health professional asks questions that enable the person to identify what has changed and what feelings, thoughts and emotions the changes are triggering within him or her. It is important to note that some of the person's thinking may be distorted because of his or her low self-esteem, and irrational beliefs may need to be sensitively dispelled, but only once the person has told you his or her story. In telling the story, people hear themselves and many times this process assists them to identify the key issues with which they are struggling and sometimes they discover ways they want to effect change. It is helpful to highlight the strengths within the people's story, but not until they know that you have really heard and understood their situation.

'*Think*' means to locate what people can/want to do about their situation. When the health professional begins to get a sense of the person's concerns they can then explore them together. After locating underlying problems/issues work together to think about possible ways in which these issues may be handled. The health professional can ask the person: 'What would you like to do about . . . ? What have you tried in the past? What is feasible? What might the consequences be? What would be the simplest and best action to move you forward?' You will find that you have helped build his or her capacity.

'*Act*' requires the health professional and person to develop a collaborative goal that can be acted on. Once the health professionals have worked with the person to identify the issue, their instinct may be to try to solve the problem. But instead of trying to fix the problem, it is important that the health professionals validate the person's feelings and their capacity to deal with the issue(s). Continue to ask questions that will lead the individual to identify possible solutions and thought-through plans of action that consider the likely outcomes of intended actions (van Loon & Kralik 2005a, 2005b, 2007). Then encourage the person to take the action(s) that will give the best result for the least effort. The fastest movement towards transition occurs when the person is able to choose his or her actions based on well thought-out and thorough reflection.

Action as the catalyst in transition

'Look, think, act' is the working process of transition. Considered and thoughtful action creates transitional processes that move people forward with life, so action is an important aspect of the 'look, think, act' process. When people only 'look' and 'think' they make little or slow progress because movement is directly correlated to a well thought-out, thorough and planned action. There is a risk involved in action so it can be easier to choose the safe option of doing nothing. Additionally, illness can make taking action difficult particularly when the person does not feel well or cannot muster the motivation and/or enthusiasm to move on.

The purpose of action is to put together practical solutions that facilitate the (re)shaping of one's future. Creating action plans can be difficult but actually enacting those plans is the most arduous aspect of the process. It will help if health professionals encourage the person to begin with something small. Actions that achieve their anticipated outcome become internal motivators that empower the person to continue with further action on the plan. With continued success the person's confidence to try new things develops, and courage and motivation grow.

Conclusion

Transition is not just another word for change (Bridges 2004), but rather the psychological processes involved in adapting to the change event or disruption. Transition is the movement and adaptation to change, rather than a return to a pre-existing state. Bridges (2004, p. 11) states that 'every transition begins with an ending,' meaning that people have to let go of familiar ways of being in the world that define who they are. This is particularly important for health professionals who are most often supporting people through forced disruption such as illness (Kralik 2002). Transitional processes require time as people gradually disengage from old habits and behaviours and ways of defining self. This represents a profound departure from the medical model of problematising the disease, so health professionals can work with people to assist them identify changes forced by illness and seek new possibilities from these experiences. We do not argue that the biomedical discourse is inappropriate or should be replaced. On the contrary, we accept that biomedical discourses focus on achieving specific health outcomes; rather we argue that a health-promoting discourse leaves room to acknowledge the impact transition has on the person's well-being. Understanding transition enables health professionals to move beyond the biomedical disease orientation to illness experiences towards a more holistic approach to the provision of care (Kralik *et al.* 1997; Kralik 2002).

Further research is required to enhance our understanding of transition. Gaps in transition research relate to gendered responses to change events, the transitional experiences during an acute episode of illness and the differences in transitions across the lifespan. Additionally, we need more information on the most appropriate activities/interventions to be provided at each phase of transition and how to facilitate the 'letting go' and 'holding on' tasks of the 'Limbo' phase.

Health professionals assist people to navigate transitions (LeVasseur 2002) as illness and change disrupt lives. Transition is a process that occurs when the person's actions and behaviours are in response to disruptive change events such as chronic illness. These actions must work toward understanding one's place in the disturbed social landscape. Learning to live with chronic illness is an ongoing complex and personal process that can take a long time. The experience of illness is constantly changing and new challenges are being generated. Over time and with the support of health professionals who use sensitive listening and thoughtful conversation, the person who is experiencing the disruption of long-term illness can locate a sense of a coherent and continuous self in a changing world. As life becomes more familiar and predictable, the person regains a sense of ordinariness that integrates aspects of the old self with which the person can forge new beginnings.

References

Arman, M., Rehnsfeldt, A. (2003) The hidden suffering among breast cancer patients: a qualitative metasynthesis. *Qualitative Health Research* **13**(4): 510–527.

Bailey, L. (1999) Refracted selves? A study of changes in self-identity in the transition to motherhood. *Sociology* **33**(2): 335–352.

Banister, E. (1999) Women's midlife experience of their changing bodies. *Qualitative Health Research* **9**(4): 520–537.

Becker, G. (1997) *Disrupted Lives: How People Create Meaning in a Chaotic World*. University of California Press: Berkley, CA.

Boeije, H., Duijnsteeb, M., Grypdonckb, M., Pool, A. (2002) Encountering the downward phase: biographical work in people with multiple sclerosis living at home. *Social Science and Medicine* **55**(6): 881–893.

Bridges, W. (2004) *Transitions: Making Sense of Life's Changes*. Da Capo Press: Cambridge, MA.

Brouwer-Dudokdewit, A., Savenije, A., Zoeteweij, M., Maat-Kievit, A., Tibben, A. (2002) A hereditary disorder in the family and the family life cycle: Huntington disease as a paradigm. *Family Process* **41**(4): 677–692.

Brudenell, I. (1996) A grounded theory of balancing alcohol recovery and pregnancy. *Western Journal of Nursing Research* **18**(4): 429–440.

Cantanzaro, M. (1990) Transitions in midlife adults with long-term illness. *Holistic Nurse Practitioner* **4**(3): 65–73.

Chick, N., Meleis, A. (1986) Transitions: a nursing concern. In: Chinn, P.L. (ed.) *Nursing Research Methodology: Issues and Implementation*, Chapter 18. Aspen: Rockville, MD, pp. 237–257.

Cranton, P. (1996) *Professional Development as Transformative Learning*. Jossey-Bass: San Francisco, CA, pp. 75–117.

Draper, J. (2003) Men's passage to fatherhood: an analysis of the contemporary relevance of transition theory. *Nursing Inquiry* **10**(1): 66–77.

Elmberger, E., Bolund, C., Lützén, K. (2002) Men with cancer: changes in attempts to master the self-image as a man and as a parent. *Cancer Nursing* **25**(6): 477–485.

Forss, A., Tishelman, C., Widmark, C., Sachs, L. (2004) Women's experiences of cervical cellular changes: an unintentional transition from health to liminality. *Sociology of Health and Illness* **26**(3): 306–325.

Fraser, C. (1999) The experience of transition for a daughter caregiver of a stroke survivor. *Journal of Neuroscience Nursing* **31**(1): 9–16.

Froggatt, K. (1997) Signposts on the journey: the place of ritual in spiritual care. *International Journal of Palliative Nursing* 3(1): 42–46.

Glacken, M., Bolund, C., Lutzen, K. (2002) Men with hepatitis C: a man and as a parent. *Cancer Nursing* 25(6): 477–485.

Glacken, M., Kernohan, G., Coates, V. (2001) Diagnosed with hepatitis C: a descriptive exploratory study. *International Journal of Nursing Studies* 38(1): 107–116.

Gwilliam, B., Bailey, C. (2001) The nature of terminal malignant bowel obstruction and its impact on patients with advanced cancer. *International Journal of Palliative Nursing* 7(10): 474–476.

Hilton, E. (2002) The meaning of stroke in elderly women: a phenomenological investigation. *Journal of Gerontological Nursing* 28(7): 19–26.

Kralik, D. (2002) The quest for ordinariness: transition experienced by midlife women living with chronic illness. *Journal of Advanced Nursing* 39(2): 146–154.

Kralik, D., Koch, T., Eastwood, S. (2003) The salience of the body: transition in sexual self-identity for women living with multiple sclerosis. *Journal of Advanced Nursing* 42(1): 11–20.

Kralik, D., Koch, T., Wotton, K. (1997) Engagement and detachment: understanding patients' experiences with nursing. *Journal of Advanced Nursing* 26(2): 399–407.

Kralik, D., van Loon, A.M., Visentin, K. (2006a) Reflection, reconciling and resilience in the chronic illness experience. *Educational Action Research* 14(2): 187–201.

Kralik, D., van Loon, A.M., Telford, K. (2006b) *Transition in Chronic Illness, Booklet: Series No. 11 Understanding Transition*. RDNS Australian Research Council: Adelaide, funded http://www.rdns.org.au/research_unit/documents/Booklet%2011%20-%20Understanding%20Transition.pdf (accessed in 2006).

Kralik, D., Visentin, K., van Loon, A. (2006c) Transition: a literature review. *Journal of Advanced Nursing* 55(3): 320–329.

Kralik, D., Seymour, L., Eastwood, S., Koch, T. (2007) Managing the self: living with an indwelling urinary catheter. *Journal of Nursing and Healthcare of Chronic Illness* 16(7b): 177–185.

LeVasseur, J. (2002) A phenomenological study of the art of nursing: experiencing the turn. *Advances in Nursing Science* 24(4): 14–26.

Lexico (2005) http://dictionary.reference.com/search?q=transition (accessed 20 May 2005).

van Loon, A.M., Kralik, D. (2005a) *Reclaiming Myself after Child Sexual Abuse*. Royal District Nursing Service Foundation Research Unit, Catherine House Inc., Alcohol Education and Rehabilitation Foundation: Adelaide. http://www.rdns.org.au/research_unit/documents/Reclaiming_Myself_Resource.pdf (accessed 2006).

van Loon, A.M., Kralik, D. (2005b) *Facilitating Transition after Child Sexual Abuse*. Royal District Nursing Service Foundation Research Unit, Catherine House Inc., Alcohol Education and Rehabilitation Foundation: Adelaide. http://www.rdns.org.au/research_unit/documents/Facilitating_Transition_Resource.pdf (accessed 2006).

van Loon, A.M., Kralik, D. (2006) Capacity building process for women with a history of child sexual abuse. *Australian Journal of Primary Health Care* 12(2): 167–176.

van Loon, A.M., Kralik, D. (2007) Facilitating transition via group work with survivors of child sexual abuse. In: Megan, J. (ed.) *Child Sexual Abuse: Issues and Challenges*. Nova Publications: Oxford.

Loveys, B. (1990) Transitions in chronic illness: the at-risk role. *Holistic Nursing Practice* 4: 45–64.

Luborsky, M. (1994) The retirement process: making the person and cultural meanings malleable. *Medical Anthropology Quarterly* **8**(4): 411–429.

Mann, R., Abercrombie, P., DeJoseph, J., Norbeck, J., Smith, R. (1999) The personal experience of pregnancy for African-American women. *Journal of Transcultural Nursing* **10**(4): 297–305.

Martin-McDonald, K., Biernoff, D. (2002) Initiation into a dialysis-dependent life: an examination of rites of passage . . . including commentary by Frauman AC with author response. *Nephrology Nursing Journal* **29**(4): 347–353.

McAdams, D., Josselson, R., Lieblich, A. (2001) *Turns in the Road: Narrative Studies of Lives in Transition*. American Psychological Association: Washington DC, USA.

Meleis, A., Sawyer, L., Im, E.-O., Hilfinger Messias, D., Schumacher, K. (2000) Experiencing transitions: an emerging middle-range theory. *Advances in Nursing Science* **23**(1): 12–28.

Meleis, A., Trangenstein, P. (1994) Facilitating transitions: redefinition of the nursing mission. *Nursing Outlook* **42**(6): 255–259.

Mezirow, J. (2000) *Learning as Transformation: Critical Perspectives on a Theory in Progress*. Jossey Bass: San Francisco, CA.

Miller, T. (2000) Losing the plot: narrative construction and longitudinal childbirth research. *Qualitative Health Research* **10**(3): 309–323.

Montenko, A., Greenberg, S. (1995) Reframing dependence in old age: a positive transition for families. *Social Work* **40**(3): 382–390.

Neil, J., Barrell, L. (1998) Transition theory and its relevance to patients with chronic wounds. *Rehabilitation Nursing* **23**(6): 295–299.

Nelson, A. (2003) Transition to motherhood. *Journal of Obstetric, Gynecologic, and Neonatal Nursing* **32**(4): 465–477.

Orlanda, F. (2001) Participatory (action) research in social theory: origin and challenges. In: Reason, P., Bradbury, H. (eds) *Handbook of Action Research*. Sage: London, pp. 27–37.

Paterson, B. (2001) The shifting perspectives model of chronic illness. *Journal of Nursing Scholarship* **33**(1): 21–26.

Paterson, B. (2003) The koala has claws: applications of the shifting perspectives model in research of chronic illness. *Qualitative Health Research* **13**(7): 987–994.

Powell-Cope, G. (1995) The experiences of gay couples affected by HIV infection. *Qualitative Health Research* **5**(1): 36–62.

Reason, P., Bradbury, H. (2001) Inquiry and participation in search of a world worthy of human aspiration. In: Reason, P., Bradbury, H. (eds) *Handbook of Action Research*. Sage: London, pp. 1–14.

Rossen, E. (1998) *Older women in relocation transition*. PhD Thesis, University of Illinois at Chicago, Health Sciences Center.

Sawyer, L. (1999) Engaged mothering: the transition to motherhood for a group of African American women. *Journal of Transcultural Nursing* **10**(1): 14–21.

Schumacher, K., Meleis, A. (1994) Transitions: a central concept in nursing. *IMAGE: Journal of Nursing Scholarship* **26**(2): 119–127.

Selder, F. (1989) Life transition theory: the resolution of uncertainty. *Nursing and Health Care* **10**(8): 437–451.

Shaul, M. (1997) Transitions in chronic illness: rheumatoid arthritis in women. *Rehabilitation Nursing* **22**(4): 199–205.

Sheehy, G. (1977) *Passages Predictable: Crisis of Adult Life*. Bantam Books: Toronto.

Skarsater, I., Dencker, K., Bergbom, I., Haggstrom, L., Fridlund, B. (2003) Women's conceptions of coping with major depression in daily life: a qualitative, salutogenic approach. *Issues in Mental Health Nursing* **24**: 419–439.

Stringer, E. (1996) *Action Research*. Sage: CA.

Stringer, E. (1999) *Action Research*, 2nd edition. Sage: CA.

Stringer, E., Genat, W. (2004) *Action Research in Health*. Pearson Merril Prentice Hall: Upper Saddle Creek, NJ.

Telford, K., Kralik, D., Koch, T. (2006) Acceptance and denial: implications for people adapting to chronic illness: literature review. *Journal of Advanced Nursing* **55**(4): 457–464.

Torosyan, R. (2007) *Teaching for Transformation: Integrative Learning, Consciousness Development and Critical Reflection*. Unpublished manuscript. http://www.faculty.fairfield.edu/rtorosyan/ (accessed 26 December 2008).

Turner, V. (1969) *The Ritual Process: Structure and Anti-structure*. Penguin: Middlesex.

Vaartio, H., Kiviniemi, K., Suominen, T. (2003) Men's experiences and their resources from cancer diagnosis to recovery. *European Journal of Oncology Nursing* **7**(3): 182–190.

Van Gennep, A. (1960) *The Rites of Passage*. Routledge & Kegan Paul: London.

Wadsworth, Y. (1991) *Principles for Participatory Action Research. Everyday Evaluation on the Run*. Action Research Issues Association : Melbourne.

Wadsworth, Y. (1998) *What Is Participatory Action Research? Action Research Resources*. http://www.scu.edu.au/schools/gcm/ar/ari/p-ywadsworth98 (accessed 2 September 2007).

White, K. (1995) The transition from victim to victor: application of the theory of mastery. *Journal of Psychosocial Nursing and Mental Health Services* **33**(8): 41–44.

White, A. (2003) Interactions between nurses and men admitted with chest pain. *European Journal of Cardiovascular Nursing* **2**(1): 47–55.

Williamson, G., Prosser, S. (2002) Action research: politics, ethics and participation. *Journal of Advanced Nursing* **40**(5): 587–593.

Young, B., Dixon-Woods, M., Findlay, M., Heney, D. (2002) Parenting in a crisis: conceptualising mothers of children with cancer. *Social Science and Medicine* **55**(10): 1835–1847.

Young-Eisendrath, P. (1996) *The Resilient Spirit: Transforming into Insight and Renewal*. Da Capo Press: New York, NY.

3. *Translating Chronic Illness Research Across the Lifespan*

Marit Kirkevold

Introduction

Chronic illness[1] is one of the leading health-related challenges across the world. During the last 30 years, chronic illness research has exploded, as illustrated by its progressive listing in databases. In 1970, no articles were indexed with the key word *chronic disease* in the CINAHL database. In 1980, there were two articles with this keyword. By 1990, there were 144, by 2000 there were 701 and by 2007 there were 2162 articles indexed with this keyword. By November 2008, a search in this database generated a total of 15,858 'hits'. Similar patterns are found in other relevant databases as well. Obviously, reviewing this research critically, with the purpose of translating it into practical measures that may improve the situation for affected individuals and groups and prevent chronic illness whenever possible, is an enormous challenge.

Chronic illness occurs across the lifespan of a person. An increasing number of people grow up to be adults with a chronic illness, because children who would have in earlier years succumbed to their disease are increasingly surviving into adulthood. Similarly, people who would previously experience significantly shortened lifespans due to chronic disease are experiencing increasing longevity due to improved disease management. Diseases such as haemophilia and cystic fibrosis are examples of such cases. A new field of study is advanced age and the management of these diseases.

Chronic illness is, by definition, a disease with a prolonged trajectory. Although there is no universal consensus about the definition, it is common to apply the

---

[1] The terms *chronic disease* and *chronic illness* are frequently used as synonyms, but have also been differentiated theoretically (see e.g. Kleinman, 1988). In this chapter *chronic illness* is the preferred term, in line with Kleinman, and used to incorporate the experienced impact of the disease on the life of the persons involved. However, in most databases classifying chronic illness research, the established term keyword is *chronic disease*, which makes retrieval of relevant research a challenge.

term if the health condition lasts for at least 6 months and impacts on the life and functioning of the ill individual, requiring monitoring and the implementation of specific management measures (Rolland 1987). In many instances, people must live with a chronic illness for many years, sometimes throughout their lives. A chronic disease may be present at birth or may occur at any time throughout the lifespan. Depending on the specific disease, it may occur abruptly and have a dramatic and downward course, it may develop slowly and have a more or less continuous and stable course or it may have an unpredictable course with episodic flare-ups (Rolland 1987; Berg & Upchurch 2007). The impact may vary from being minor to incapacitating, and it may be life-shortening to a lesser or larger degree (Rolland 1987). The character of the illness, then, is a significant factor in terms of the consequences it has for the life of the ill person and his or her family (Berg & Upchurch 2007). So far, much of the research conducted has concentrated on identifying the causes and effective treatment and has explored how different chronic illnesses impact on the lives of the affected persons and/or their families.

Chronic illness may impact people differently, depending on which stage of the lifespan the person is in, as well as where in the life cycle the family finds itself (Rolland 1987; Berg & Upchurch 2007). Research has increasingly addressed this issue. In particular, researchers have been concerned with the impact of chronic disease in childhood and adolescence, both in terms of how the disease has impacted on the child or adolescent himself or herself and how chronic illness has impacted on families having a chronically ill child or adolescent (Miles & Holditch-Davis 2003). Chronic illness research has also documented the impact of chronic illness in other phases throughout the lifespan, particularly in young and middle adulthood (Miles & Holditch-Davis 2003). Research has focused less on chronic illness, with particular reference to old age (Putnam 2002).

Despite these findings, an explicit and theoretically informed lifespan approach to chronic illness research has been quite limited. A recent search (conducted in November 2008) generated 299 articles in MEDLINE, 90 articles in Sociological Abstracts, 55 articles in CINAHL and 33 articles in Psych Info, using the key words *chronic disease, life cycle, life course, lifespan* and *human development* in various combinations. A large part of this research focused on factors contributing to the development of chronic illness. Recent advances in life course epidemiology have generated new insights into the impact of genetic factors, environmental factors and lifestyle factors on the development and course of chronic illness (Gluckman *et al.* 2007). Similar lines of research have focused on sociological aspects of chronic illness, documenting the cumulative disadvantage of particular segments of populations, that is, people of ethnic minorities, people with a low socio-economic status, users of addictive substances, etc. (Smith 2007). This prospective population-focused research is highly relevant in terms of developing health-care policies that may prevent the development of chronic disease. It is less relevant, however, for individuals and families already living with chronic illness, which is the focus of this chapter.

Given the fact that chronic illness occurs across the lifespan and is a condition that persists over time, a human developmental perspective on chronic illness

38

would seem highly relevant. Surprisingly, this focus has received relatively scant attention from chronic illness researchers. So far, it has primarily been addressed by researchers interested in chronic illnesses in childhood and adolescence (Miles & Holditch-Davis 2003), whereas the application of an explicit human development perspective in the last part of the lifespan or across the lifespan is severely understudied. The goal of this chapter is to highlight the relevance of a developmental perspective on chronic illness in order to understand how chronic illness and human development interact to impact on the life of individuals and families across the lifespan. Initially, a review of the central tenets of the human development perspective is provided. This is followed by a brief review of the current state of affairs with regard to applying a lifespan developmental perspective in chronic illness research. Finally, examples of chronic illness research informed by a lifespan developmental perspective are reviewed. In this chapter, research focusing on cystic fibrosis (CF) is chosen to exemplify a chronic illness that 'follows' the person from birth to death thereby impacting on the whole lifespan of the individual. Dementia is the second selected example. This increasingly prevalent disease, particularly, though not exclusively, associated with old age, highlights specific challenges related to the interaction of ageing and chronic illness in advanced age. Particular attention is given to research aimed at testing developmentally appropriate interventions in order to stimulate future research that may support individuals and their significant others to integrate chronic illness with other developmental tasks and transitions across the lifespan.

Human development across the lifespan

Human development is described as a theoretical orientation or perspective that encompasses a number of theoretical foci and perspectives (Baltes *et al*. 1980). Traditionally, it has been divided into biological development and maturation, psychological development and social development (Weekes 1995). *Biological development* refers to the organism's growth and maturation (Baltes *et al*. 1980) and is usually thought of in terms of increased differentiation at the cellular, organ, organ system and bodily levels leading to qualitatively different, irreversible, end state-oriented and universal patterns of change such as that occurring in muscular–skeletal strength and coordination and with regard to cognitive abilities (Baltes *et al*. 1980). Biological growth and maturation occur predominantly in the early phases of life, notably through childhood and adolescence. Biological ageing (which is usually associated with loss rather than growth and development) is said to begin around 25 years of age and progresses steadily towards death. Recent research has found a more multidimensional and multi-linear pattern of biological development, in which development at all ages entails both gains and losses (Baltes 1987).

Psychological development refers to the cognitive and emotional changes that occur over the lifespan (Baltes *et al*. 1980). It encompasses a broad range of psycho-physiological processes involved in cognitive and emotional development including problem-solving, moral understanding, conceptual understanding, language acquisition, personality, self-concept and identity formation (Baltes *et al.* 1980). Psychological development has traditionally been thought of as progressing through several stages associated with specific developmental tasks (Baltes *et al.* 1980). Influential theories have been, among others, that of Piaget (2002) on cognitive development in childhood and of E. H. Erikson (1982) and Erikson *et al.* (1986) on psychosocial development across the lifespan. The latter divides the lifespan into eight stages, each of which encompasses a developmental crisis that the individual must resolve to achieve increasing personal maturity and wisdom. Each stage presents the individual with two opposing 'poles'. The task is to attain the positive developmental goal. The individual should either accomplish the developmental task positively and move towards greater psychosocial maturity and strength or else must move on with a developmental 'weakness' (Erikson 1964). The latter situation may impact on psychosocial well-being at the time and during the individual's subsequent development. According to this theory (Erikson 1982; Erikson *et al.* 1986), the crises in childhood are trust versus mistrust, autonomy versus shame and doubt, initiative versus guilt and industry versus inferiority. In adolescence, the crisis entails identity versus identity confusion. In adulthood, crises include intimacy versus isolation and generativity versus self-absorption and in old age integrity versus despair. When confronted with each new crisis, previous crises that have been latent may therefore be reactivated. It should be noted that this theory, in line with most of the developmental lifespan theories, is heavily influenced by Western cultural values emphasising individual autonomy. Its relevance for other cultures may therefore be questioned, an issue that has received scant attention so far.

Social development is closely related to psychological development and maturation. A central theme is socialisation, that is, the processes by which persons and groups acquire different social roles and accomplish culturally assigned social tasks and responsibilities at different phases across the life cycle (Damon & Hart 1992; Cairns *et al.* 1996). The transmission and transformation of socio-cultural values, beliefs, norms and practices across generations and social groups over time are at the heart of social development theories (Cairns *et al.* 1996). Social contextual factors impacting on interpersonal interactions between individuals and groups, including patterns of group dynamics, negotiation and conflict, are central topics. Studies of family development, social support and caregiving expectations and practices are salient health-related topics (Berg & Upchurch 2007).

Key assumptions of the lifespan developmental perspective

The idea of fixed stages and specific tasks encountered at particular times during the life course has recently been challenged as providing too simplistic and inflexible a picture of development to account for the wide variation across individuals, ages, health and social contexts (Baltes *et al.* 1980). A more flexible, pluralistic and multi-linear conception of development has therefore gained prominence (Baltes 1987). In their seminal review of human development, which is still considered an authoritative synthesis of the lifespan developmental perspective

(Rankin & Weekes 2000; Carstensen *et al.* 2003; Berg & Upchurch 2007), Baltes *et al.* (1980) argue that across the lifespan, individuals and groups are exposed to different kinds of influences that interact in a complex and multidirectional manner to determine human development. Emphasising that biological and environmental factors are closely interrelated, they introduce three classes of 'bio-cultural' influencing factors, termed *normative age-graded influences, normative history-graded influences* and *non-normative influences*.

- *Normative age-graded* influences are defined as 'biological and environmental determinants that have (in terms of onset and duration) a fairly strong relationship with chronological age' (Baltes *et al.* 1980, p. 75). Examples are biological maturation and age-graded socialisation events within the family, in relation to education and with regard to occupation. Traditional developmental theories have primarily been concerned with normative age-graded development.
- *Normative history-graded* influences are those biological and environmental determinants associated with historical time and historical contexts. 'They are normative in that they occur to most members of a given cohort (generation) in similar ways, although the events may differ for different age-cohorts living at the same time' (Baltes *et al.* 1980, p. 75). Major social changes, economic recession and war are examples of normative history-graded influences.
- *Non-normative life events* encompass biological and environmental influences that do not follow an age-graded or history-graded pattern for most individuals. Such significant life events may be the result of serious illness or accidents, death of a significant other, relocation, unemployment, divorce, etc. These are non-normative in the sense that there is wide inter-individual variation in the occurrence and pattern of such influences. They can occur at any time across the lifespan (Baltes *et al.* 1980).

The nature of human development depends on the joint impact of these influences, mediated through the developing individual. The complex interaction of these factors accounts for the inter-individual differences, the multidirectional and the multidimensional nature of human development across the lifespan (Baltes *et al.* 1980). Baltes *et al.* (1980) have summarised the multidimensional nature of human development in Figure 3.1.

In their analysis, Baltes *et al.* (1980) and Baltes (1987) hypothesise that age-graded, history-graded and non-normative influences have differential impact across the lifespan, although this has not been adequately studied. They suggest that age-graded factors have higher impact in childhood and in old age, whereas history-graded influences are particularly salient in adolescence and young adulthood. They underpin their hypothesis by the accumulated evidence within developmental psychology that childhood development has high levels of consistency and predictability. This may be accounted for by the significant impact of hereditary factors in early life. In old age, psychological ageing depends more on experiences and cohort effects than on hereditary factors. Nevertheless, the impact of biological and environmental factors increases in old age, as biological and psychological ageing take their toll (Baltes & Smith 2003).

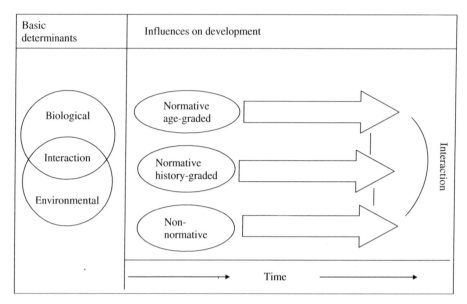

Figure 3.1 Factors impacting on human development. Source: (Baltes *et al.* 1980. Reprinted, with permission, from the *Annual Review of Psychology*, Volume 31, © 1980 by Annual Reviews [www.annualreviews.org]).

Baltes *et al.* (1980) argue that the reason for history-graded influences to have their highest impact in adolescence is that adolescence and young adulthood are the periods in which the intergenerational dialectics and the interaction between society and the individual are most salient. In these periods, much of the foundation for adulthood is established including developing an identity, completing an education, launching a career, forming an intimate relationship, establishing a family, etc. The way these significant life tasks are met is highly dependent on the socio-environmental climate, which makes significant historical events particularly salient. Non-normative influences probably increase over time because they are related to the experience of significant life events, which tend to accumulate with age (Baltes 1997; Baltes & Smith 2003).

Human development in old age

Whereas early lifespan research was primarily concerned with the first parts of life, particularly childhood and adolescence, recent advances in lifespan research has been particularly concerned with the last part of the life cycle. This is related to significant demographic changes around the world. During the last century, the lifespan has increased considerably and there has been an exponential increase in the number of old people (Baltes & Smith 2003). These changes have given rise to the notions of the 'third' and 'fourth' ages in the lifespan development literature (Baltes & Smith 2003). This differentiation of the last part of the lifespan into two separate phases is important because of the characteristic patterns of gains (growth) and losses (decline) seen in the 'young old' and the 'old old' (Baltes & Smith 2003; Carstensen *et al.* 2003).

For most people in developed nations, the third age (also referred to as 'young old' age), is usually considered to last between approximately 65 and 80 years of age. Good physical and mental health generally characterise this period, although a substantial number of people will experience the advent of one or more chronic conditions during this period. In general, older people have experienced an increase in the number of 'good' years amounting to an average of 5 years with good physical and mental health (Baltes & Smith 2003). These changes are related to better material environments, more advanced medical practice, improved economic conditions, more effective education and media systems and increased psychological resources. Accumulating research has demonstrated that the 'young old' have substantial cognitive and emotional reserves that can be used to deal with life's challenges and task. There is ample evidence, for example, that most people, at least in the developed countries, maintain their level of everyday intelligence or mental achievement until around age 70 (Baltes & Smith 2003; Löckenhoff & Carstensen 2007), some significantly longer, given the wide variations in old age. Other studies have found that culture- and practice-nurtured functioning can be maintained into the late 80s (Baltes & Smith 2003). Emotional intelligence and wisdom are also maintained, or even increased, with age. Empirical studies have consistently found that older people are at the top of all age groups with regard to these aspects.

Emotional intelligence refers to the ability to, both, understand the causes of different emotions and develop strategies to avoid emotional conflict situations or to change their negative consequences, particularly with regard to difficult life problems between people (Baltes & Smith 2003; Löckenhoff & Carstensen 2007). Wisdom refers to 'an ideal combination of mindfulness and virtue' and 'an expertise in matters of conduct, meaning and interpretation of life' (Baltes & Smith 2003, p. 126–127). A third characteristic strength of older people in their third age is their astonishing capacity of 'self-plasticity' (Baltes & Smith 2003, p. 127).

From 70 years of age, the chance of experiencing decreasing health and the presence of one or more chronic illnesses increases dramatically (Baltes & Smith 2003). At the same time, older people have great potential for adjusting to changed life conditions, including changes in illness and health. This ability encompasses people's psychological capacity to transform reality through internal adaptations and reconstructions: 'When people have to deal with an illness, they compare themselves with others who have similar or even worse illnesses. The power of plasticity of the self and the ability to transform beliefs amount to some of the best insurance policies for well-being in old age one can have' (Baltes & Smith 2003, p. 127). These particular strengths, the accumulated experiences and increased coping skills over time, are highly relevant in managing chronic illness. Unfortunately, health professionals frequently neglect the substantial expertise and coping abilities exhibited by older persons, who may have lived with chronic conditions for years (Paterson 2001; Kvigne *et al.* 2005).

In contrast to this positive side of ageing, the fourth age (or 'old old' age) presents quite a different picture. The very old approach the limits of the biological and psychological abilities. Referring to an increasing number of empirical studies, Baltes and Smith (2003) argue that in the fourth age, the cognitive potential and ability to learn decline significantly. This is partly related to the substantial increase in dementia seen in this age group; approximately 50% of all 90-year-olds suffer from dementia. However, even in the 'healthy' oldest old, new learning is severely impaired (Baltes & Smith 2003). The prolific cognitive changes seen in the very old lead to the loss of many fundamental qualities important for experiencing well-being and quality of life including intentionality, autonomy, independent living, personal identity and social connectedness – aspects closely related to the experience of human dignity (Baltes & Smith 2003).

The progressing biological and psychosocial ageing processes and the accumulation of chronic health conditions reduce the reserve capacity of the 'old old' persons, thereby moving them steadily closer to the limits of their abilities. This leads to 'chronic life strains' (i.e. multi-dysfunctionality and multi-morbidity), which is almost five times higher in this age group, compared to the 'young old' (Baltes & Smith 2003, p. 129). The authors conclude that in the fourth age 'few functions remain robust and resilient to negative change. The rate of negative change is larger if aging is superimposed by pathology' (Baltes & Smith 2003, p. 130).

Concurrent with the biological loss associated with the ageing process, the supportive and compensatory role of culture-based resources increases in significance. The material, mental, social and technological aspects of modern societies are major compensatory factors that may facilitate functioning, reduce the impact of disabilities and increase quality of life (Baltes 1997; Baltes & Smith 2003).

Despite the strong evidence of functional decline during the fourth age, Baltes and Smith (2003) do not draw a completely bleak picture of adaptability among the very old. According to their theory of selection, optimization and compensation (SOC) (Baltes 1997), older people who are able to prioritise areas of interest, activities and tasks that they can still master (selection), utilise and/or practice skills that make them able to maintain an adequate level of functioning in these areas (optimization) and/or replace strategies/skills they are no longer able to carry out with ones that they are able to master (compensation), maintain a sense of well-being and agency even when facing progressive decline. These researchers maintain that 'the art of life in old age consists of the creative search for a new usually smaller territory that is cared for with similar intensity as in the past' (Baltes & Smith 2003, p. 132). With regard to supporting people who are the 'old old' managing chronic illness, a particularly salient issue would be to identify and maintain the strengths of the person by assisting the individual to select the most important and relevant issues to direct one's coping abilities towards, maintain and optimise the person's coping strategies and skills and offer assistance and care that may maintain and compensate for decreasing functions in close collaboration with the older person and his or her significant others. Other researchers have documented that similar processes occur throughout the lifespan if the individual lifespan is perceived to be short, that is, due to life-threatening disease (Carstensen 2006) or if serious illness impacts on the physical, mental and/or psychosocial capacity of the person (Ebner *et al*. 2006).

The lifespan developmental perspective has several implications in terms of understanding the interaction between chronic illness and developmental tasks and issues across the lifespan. First, understanding the interdependence and inter-action of biological and psychosocial developmental processes is highly salient in understanding how chronic illness may create additional strains on the nor-mative age-graded developmental tasks. The advent of a chronic disease may pose a serious threat in terms of the integrity of the biological development of an individual. This seems to be particularly the case during childhood, where bio-logical growth and maturity is most prominent, and in late old age, where biological ageing imposes escalating limits on the reserve capacity of the indi-vidual. Secondly, the human development perspective underscores that the impact of chronic illness depends on history and time. The cohort perspective (i.e. the impact of normative history-graded influences) emphasises the impor-tance of integrating socio-cultural and historical perspectives into chronic illness research in order to understand how chronic illness may impact differently across generations.

The human developmental perspective, with its roots in psychology and soci-ology, has normal development and maturation as the major focus and considers chronic illness a potentially negative influencing factor. Its status as a 'non-normative' influencing factor indicates that it is not considered an expected developmental challenge across the lifespan, possibly except in the last phase of life. This may explain the lack of psychosocial preparation for handling the chronic illness repeatedly found in the chronic illness literature. Even in the latter part of the lifespan, people who abruptly become chronically ill experience a major life disruption and a subsequent demanding and prolonged adjustment process, involving changes in identity and psychosocial maturity (Kirkevold 2002). The advent of chronic illness initiates a transition that requires adaptation of all involved (Schlossberg 1981; Goodman *et al*. 2006). The human develop-mental perspective underscores that the impact of this transition depends on other life events and developmental issues concurrently important in the lives of individuals and families.

The human development perspective offers a largely optimistic view of persons' ability to deal with developmental challenges across the lifespan. Both individuals and families seem to gain increased abilities to meet challenges as they mature. Nevertheless, negative experiences early in life may inhibit human development unless successfully mastered. Unfortunately, a massive body of research docu-ments that such experiences are not equally distributed but tend to accumulate over time in socially and culturally non-privileged groups (Gluckman *et al*. 2007; Smith 2007). This highlights the importance of increased focus on social inequal-ities in health-related chronic illness research, focusing on how individuals and their families deal with chronic illness across the lifespan and how best to assist them in living well despite their health concern. At the same time, it is important to acknowledge that people who have lived with chronic illness over many years have developed considerable experience and a level of expertise in managing their conditions. This needs to be recognised and built upon in order to support well-being.

Applications of lifespan developmental perspectives in chronic illness research

During the last 20 years, the significance of applying a human developmental perspective in chronic illness research has repeatedly been stressed in relation to individuals and families. In an early review, Rankin and Weekes (2000) observed that 'a theoretical basis for understanding the impact of chronic or acute illness on the well-being of the family is not yet delineated' (p. 355). They proposed using the model of Baltes *et al.* (1980) because of its relevance in exploring 'the dynamic, integrated aspects of human functioning', which they considered particularly relevant to nursing. Reviewing selected research on families with chronically ill members in light of the selected lifespan developmental perspective, they proposed several propositions with regard to the interaction of lifespan development, chronic illness and family well-being for further study. Interestingly, the article was published without amendment a decade later (Rankin & Weekes 2000), suggesting that their cry for intensified research in this area fell on 'deaf ears' the first time around.

Taking a more circumscribed perspective, Weekes (1995) proposed that the lifespan perspective was highly relevant when studying adolescents growing up chronically ill. She saw it as a major challenge to gain increased understanding of how development occurs within the context of chronic illness in order to explicate coping approaches that may facilitate enhanced quality of life for chronically ill adolescents. Weekes applied this perspective when studying adolescents suffering from cancer.

Miles and Holditch-Davis (2003) edited a volume of the *Annual Review of Nursing Research* exclusively focusing on nursing research with children and families from a developmental science perspective. They criticised pediatric nursing research for not being based on the latest developments in relevant scientific fields, and specifically sought to 'move nursing research with children forward towards more developmentally sound knowledge of nursing practice' (p. 1). Drawing on 'developmental science', as developed by Cairns *et al.* (1996), Miles and Holditch-Davis underscored the contribution of 'developmental systems theory' in understanding human development as a complex 'interaction of biological, social, and ecological factors within and without the person over the life course' (p. 8). They emphasised longitudinal designs and person-oriented analysis (rather than variable-focused research) in order to capture individual developmental pathways and outcomes over time and in specific ecological contexts (Bronfenbrenner 1989). The general impression of the reviews in this volume is the lack of sophisticated research in this area.

Berg and Upchurch (2007) propose a new 'developmental–contextual' model of couples coping with chronic illness across the adult lifespan. Arguing that most chronic illness research has had an individual focus, studying coping over time either in the ill person or in individual family members (notably the spouse), Berg and Upchurch maintain that a dyadic or coupled perspective is necessary because coping in one partner strongly impacts on, and is impacted by, the coping of the other. They maintain, furthermore, that couples' coping with illness may vary over time, depending on the character of the illness, the nature of the marital relationship and the time in the life cycle. Focusing on dyadic appraisal, coping and adjustment over time, the authors highlight the importance of studying how similarities and differences between the spouses' appraisal, coping and adjustment interact over time and how different dyadic coping styles may facilitate or hinder adjustment to chronic illness for each partner and for the couple as such. They conclude that this is a novel area in need of intensified research.

Seen together, these publications present a united message regarding chronic illness research from a developmental lifespan perspective. Developmentally sensitive research, focusing on how chronic illness and human development interact over time in individuals across all ages, in couples and in families over the life cycle, is highly needed but is still in many ways in its infancy. Nevertheless, recent advances in theoretical perspectives on lifespan development provide promise for this to become a ripe area of research in the future. In the next section, we look at selected examples of research in order to illustrate the usefulness of applying a developmental perspective on chronic illness research in order to generate developmentally appropriate knowledge and support measures.

Supporting age-appropriate development without jeopardising the safe management of serious chronic disease: the case of cystic fibrosis

Cystic fibrosis is a progressive genetic disease without a cure. It leads to significantly shortened lifespan, though median survival rate has increased dramatically during the last 40 years, from 12 years in 1966 to more than 30 years in 2004 (CFF 2004). More than 40% of the CF population is currently above 18 years of age. CF, then, is a serious chronic illness that follows the affected individuals throughout their lives, thereby highlighting salient issues related to how to incorporate the illness-related implications with developmental issues across the lifespan.

Christian *et al.* (1999), Christian (2003) and Christian and D'Auria (2006) are among the few researchers who have systematically studied the impact of living with CF over time. They have sought to develop and test developmentally appropriate interventions intended to support the management of chronic illness, while at the same time honour the developmental needs of these individuals over time. Their research, and related studies, will be used as an example of how chronic illness research may be translated into practice, relevant insights and interventions in order to reduce the vulnerability caused by the disease and support the young individuals' own coping abilities as they develop and grow.

According to Christian and D'Auria (2006), many of the stresses that chronically ill children encounter occur within the context of coping with peer responses to their illness-related differences. Middle childhood (6–12 years) is a particularly vulnerable time because children in this age are increasingly developing a sense of self and of self-worth by comparing themselves to other children in the same age and defining themselves by the social groups to which they belong. This places children with serious chronic conditions in a vulnerable state. As observed by Christian and D'Auria (2006): 'When entering school, children with CF are challenged to meet normal developmental demands while dealing with the non-normative demands of the disease process' (p. 301). This may lead to feelings of incompetence, low self-worth and loneliness because of the physical and social limitations that the disease may cause.

To assist children manage this complex challenge, Christian and D'Auria (2006) developed an intervention based on their previous research and guided by a developmental framework (Damon & Hart 1992; Sroufe *et al.* 1996) and a social ecological perspective (Bronfenbrenner 1986). The intervention aimed at improving the psychosocial adjustment and the functional and physiologic health of children with CF. The 'Building Life-skills' intervention was an educational problem-solving and social skills intervention designed to help children aged 8–12 to deal with specific problems encountered during middle childhood. Consisting of four intervention modules, it focused on improving the child's understanding of CF and daily disease management, explaining CF-related differences to peers, dealing with teasing and keeping up with peers during physical activity. The intervention was administered as one individually tailored session, carried out in the child's at-home session, and three group sessions. The individual session was geared towards assisting the child make sense of the CF diagnosis and construct his or her own personal history of CF. Developmentally appropriate individualised content was delivered about physiological and functional health changes, adherence to treatment and self-care, using age-adjusted learning tools such as electronic learning materials and colourful notebooks. The individual session was foundational for the group sessions, which focused on explaining CF-related differences to peers, dealing with teasing and keeping up with peers during physical activity. Group interactions involved a combination of educational content, fun activities and getting-to-know-you activities, ending with a social pizza party (Christian & D'Auria 2006). This study, which applied a two-group, experimental, repeated measures design, randomised children with CF into two groups of 58 participants each. The participants were followed up for 9 months. (For more details about the study, see Christian & D'Auria 2006.)

The intervention showed significant differences between the intervention and control groups with regard to perceived impact of the illness on quality of life, loneliness and global self-worth. These effects remained over time. There were no significant effects on functional and physiological health, or on self-competence and peer support, although the latter two changed significantly over time in both groups. The authors concluded that the intervention succeeded in teaching children with CF to manage the demands of chronic illness in the social context of their everyday lives thereby increasing their quality of life. The intervention provided the participants with the opportunity to improve their social skills thereby improving peer relations as well as establishing a CF peer group. This led to significant improvements in the alleviation of loneliness and in global self-worth and self-competence over time, which are developmentally significant in this age group (Christian & D'Auria 2006).

Being a progressive disorder, the disease process of CF will eventually lead to an end stage in which the individual's physiologic state is precarious and life threatening. For most CF patients, this will occur during late adolescence or young adulthood (Christian *et al*. 1999). The most common life-threatening complication of CF is related to lung insufficiency (Christian *et al*. 1999). In recent years, lung transplantation has become the most effective treatment of choice. This creates a most significant non-normative challenge for young people in which they will have to make a decision whether or not to be put on 'the list' (i.e. being formally screened and put on the list for persons awaiting a suitable lung donor for a lung transplantation).

Only a few studies (Christian *et al*. 1999; Macdonald 2006) have explored how adolescents and young adults experience this period. In a qualitative case study of the deliberations and choices made by one adolescent over a period of 1 year, Christian *et al*. (1999) found that the decision about when to become a 'lung transplant candidate' was not only a consequence of the illness progression. Rather, it was strongly impacted by age-related developmental needs, such as maintaining a life in which peer relationships and meaningful activities (i.e. continuing his studies) were essential elements. The participant exerted his or her independence by maintaining the right to make decisions on his or her own behalf with regard to evaluating the consequences of balancing the risk-taking behaviour of delaying 'being put on the list' with the need to avoid becoming 'listed' too late, thereby missing the 'therapeutic window' when a lung transplant is still medically feasible. Christian *et al*. (1999) use this case study to highlight the interaction between the developmental needs and abilities of adolescents and the demands with regard to managing the requirements of the disease. The case study illustrates how adolescents must evaluate their situation and make complex decisions on serious health and life problems. The authors stress the importance of health-care professionals supporting adolescents and young adults and their close and worried relatives in negotiating a balance between illness-related needs and developmental needs.

In a similar study from the United Kingdom, Macdonald (2006) conducted in-depth qualitative interviews with eight persons suffering from CF, four awaiting lung transplantation and four who had been through lung transplantation. The participants, five men and three women aged 19–40 years, described going through a demanding process characterised by experiences of 'displacement' from their 'normal life' created by being recommended to consider lung transplantation, a recommendation that led to surprise and anger and a need for reassessment of oneself and one's illness. The process of being 'listed' entailed a process of clinical scrutiny associated with emotional upheaval and 'disorder'. Finally, becoming a lung transplant candidate led to a 'life in limbo' where the CF patient, to a large extent, experienced putting 'life on hold' in order to be prepared and ready should the 'peeper' go off (Macdonald 2006).

Unlike the studies of Christian *et al*. (1999) and Christian and D'Auria (2006), Macdonald did not analyse her data from a developmental perspective, although the age of the participants ranged from 19 to 40, which covers adolescence, young adulthood and even middle age. Seen from a developmental perspective, having one's life 'put on hold' is experienced as very dramatic in adolescence and early adulthood because of the major transitions occurring during this time including completing an education, establishing intimate relationships and pursuing a career. Moving towards middle adulthood, developmental concerns related to participating in meaningful productive and socially relevant activities are more in focus. Some may be in a position where they are responsible for the care of others, for example, a partner or children generating other concerns and worries.

Seen together, these studies illuminate the potential of the developmental lifespan perspective in chronic illness. In a recent review, Christian (2003) uncovered that although developmental perspectives had been applied in a number of studies of CF, more research is needed to evolve developmentally appropriate interventions across the whole lifespan of CF patients and their families to support chronic illness management while at the same time facilitating human development.

Chronic illness in old age: providing developmentally appropriate integrity-promoting care to persons suffering from dementia

Few studies have focused on human development in relation to chronic illness in the last phase of the lifespan. An exception is the work of Astrid Nordberg and colleagues in Umeå, Sweden. In a series of studies focusing on persons suffering from dementia, this research group has applied the developmental theory of EH Erikson (1982) and Erikson *et al.* (1986) to explore interactions between care-dependent patients and professional carers and to develop interventions that may support the integrity of this vulnerable group of patients.

In a study conducted within the long-term ward setting, Kihlgren (1992) and Kihlgren *et al.* (1993, 1996) explored the effect on patient–nurse interactions of a training programme for staff that was directed towards strengthening the integrity of old persons with dementia. The intervention, entitled 'Integrity-promoting care', was based on EH Erikson and J Erikson's theory of eight stages of man (1982, 1986). The basic assumptions of the study were that the experience of wholeness and meaning is essential to 'form one's daily life and make it function' (Kihlgren 1992, p. 9) and that this experience is severely disturbed as a consequence of the degenerative cognitive changes following dementia. Erikson's theory posits that old persons are in the last (eighth) stage of psychosocial development and have to look back on life and forward towards death. In this stage, they can either accept life as it turned out or be filled with grief and despair. The positive resolution leads to an experience of wholeness and meaning, called *integrity* (Erikson & Erikson 1981; Erikson *et al.* 1986). The ability to achieve integrity is severely disabled by impaired memory. Consequently, persons with dementia need support from the social environment to maintain their history.

The resolution of crises during a person's life cycle leaves its mark on the developing person in terms of strengths (virtues) or weaknesses (antipathic), depending on whether the solutions were positive or negative (Kihlgren 1992). These emerging qualities of the person impact on the person's expectations and daily interactions with his or her surroundings. All human beings need a supporting environment to maintain hope, will, purpose, competence, fidelity, love, care and wisdom, which are the strengths or virtues resulting from positive resolution of the developmental crises across life (Erikson 1982; Kihlgren 1992). However, because of the progressive impairments of sensory, perceptual and cognitive processes ensuing from dementia, these patients are becoming particularly vulnerable and increasingly dependent on carers to promote the positive poles of the developmental crises. This involves developing an adjusted 'milieu' that may foster the strengths (virtues) of the person, while refraining from exacerbating the weaknesses (Kihlgren 1992). Based on the theoretical ideas of EH Erikson and J Erikson, Kihlgren (1992) and Kihlgren *et al.* (1993, 1996) developed a staff developmental programme intended to assist the long-term staff in providing 'integrity-promoting care' to patients suffering from moderate to severe dementia.

The basic principle of integrity-promoting care was intended for the staff to promote the experience of wholeness and meaning in patients through the care provided. Wholeness and meaning was interpreted to be present if the patients exhibited behaviours indicative of trust, autonomy, initiative, industry, identity, intimacy, generativity and integrity, which in turn led to the disclosure of positive qualities of their personality, that is, the strengths of hope, will, purpose, competence, fidelity, love, care and wisdom (Kihlgren 1992, p. 33). In concrete terms, integrity-promoting care entailed elements such as greeting and orienting the patient before acting, using the person's first name, encouraging the patient to participate in decisions and activities, giving the person the opportunity to see him/herself in the mirror, asking for the patient's opinions and wishes and providing time to respond before proceeding. By providing additional time, using body contact to console, communicating at 'face height' and expressing confidence and respect in the patient, a positive atmosphere was created (Kihlgren 1992; Kihlgren *et al.* 1993).

The intervention study was carried out in one intervention ward (IW) with 28 patients suffering from moderate to serious dementia and one control ward (CW) of 30 patients with similar conditions in two different long-term institutions. The wards were staffed with 0.69 and 0.73 personnel per bed, respectively. The staff in the IW received a 1-week course in integrity-promoting care followed by a 3-month follow-up supervision period. Data were collected using observations of physical environment and routines, questionnaires to staff, video-recordings of patient–staff interactions, measurement of psychological, biochemical and functional abilities of the patients, and interviews with staff (for details, see Kihlgren *et al.* 1996).

The researchers (Kihlgren 1992; Kihlgren *et al.* 1993, 1996) found that the integrity-promoting care improved the quality of the interactions and communication between staff and patients (Kihlgren *et al.* 1993). Applying neurochemical and neurophysiological parameters, they found less deterioration in the intervention group compared to the controls. They also found evidence of improved motor and social ability, somewhat better intellectual ability, more alertness and reduced signs of depression (Kihlgren 1992). The patients exhibited more autonomy and initiative (Kihlgren *et al*. 1996). They also found evidence that patients made efforts to change negative interactions with caregivers into positive ones and showed better conversational competence than expected (e.g. in terms of providing praise and critique to caregivers). Several patients in the intervention group showed increased appetite and gained weight (Kihlgren 1992).

Interpreting their findings in light of Erikson's theory, Kihlgren *et al*. (1996) suggested that the atmosphere that the staff was able to create and the integrity-promoting interactions that ensued supported the patients in utilising their remaining cognitive, emotional and physical abilities to their fullest. As a consequence of the cognitive changes of their condition, persons with dementia are more susceptible to social stress (Kihlgren 1992). By creating an integrity-promoting atmosphere, in which the interactions and care were directed towards supporting the positive poles in the psychosocial, the positive qualities of their personality became more evident. Although still exceedingly difficult, the success in accomplishing this made it easier for the staff to establish a relationship based on mutuality and collaboration, increasing the staff's experiences of meaning and fulfilment in their work (Kihlgren *et al*. 1993, 1996).

The findings in the studies reviewed above extend a number of other studies guided by Erikson's theory, conducted by the same research group. For example, existential dimensions of eating among persons with dementia were explored by Norberg and Sandman (1988) and Hallberg (1990). Ekman *et al*. (1995) found that carers who were able to communicate with bilingual persons with dementia in their mother tongue were more successful in promoting their integrity. In a recently published study (Mamhidir *et al*. 2007), integrity-promoting care was found to be associated with increased weight among persons with dementia. Unfortunately, so far this line of research has not been replicated or extended by other research groups. It remains one of few published examples with the human developmental perspective explicitly applied when attempting to design developmentally appropriate interventions among old persons suffering from chronic illness.

Conclusions and implications

Despite its obvious relevance and repeated calls for strengthening this line of research during the last 20 years, chronic illness research has so far largely neglected a lifespan developmental perspective. This may be due to the complex methodological and theoretical challenges that are involved in conducting this kind of research. Developmental research is longitudinal in nature, although it may focus on a shorter or longer part of the lifespan (Baltes 1997; Berg & Upchurch 2007). It must incorporate the multidimensionality, multi-directionality and flexibility of human development, as described in recent theoretical developments (Baltes *et al*. 1980; Baltes 1997). Research is needed both on 'micro-development' evolving in daily interactions within a circumscribed period of time (Kihlgren *et al*. 1996; Berg & Upchurch 2007) and on development at a more general overarching level across the lifespan. Because human development is ecological in nature, developmental research needs to go beyond focusing on individuals to looking at how human development occurs concurrently in individuals and groups who are closely connected, such as children and their parents, couples, siblings and close friends (Rolland 1987; Rankin & Weekes 2000; Miles & Holditch-Davis 2003).

The nature and development of the chronic condition itself cannot be neglected in developmentally sensitive chronic illness research. Chronic illness is an exceedingly complex phenomenon with huge variations in terms of onset, course, consequences and impact of the ill persons and those close to them (Berg & Upchurch 2007). Taking the longitudinal nature of chronic illness into account when studying the interaction of human development and being chronically ill across the lifespan may greatly increase our understanding. The nature of the transitions and the adaptation processes that are required will depend on both the chronic illness itself – where in the lifespan the individual and family members find themselves – and on other salient issues present in the lives of those involved (Goodman *et al.* 2006). Although methodologically challenging, such research may facilitate designing developmentally appropriate interventions across the lifespan thereby improving the support provided to individuals and families struggling to live their lives to the fullest despite their long-term health condition.

References

Baltes, P.B. (1987) Theoretical proposition of life-span developmental psychology: on the dynamics between growth and decline. *Developmental Psychology* **23**(5): 611–626.

Baltes, P.B. (1997) On the incomplete architecture of human ontogeny. Selection, optimization, and compensation as foundation of developmental theory. *American Psychologist* **52**(4): 366–380.

Baltes, P.B., Reese, H.W., Lipsitt, L.P. (1980) Life-span developmental psychology. *Annual Reviews in Psychology* **31**: 65–110.

Baltes, P.R., Smith, J. (2003) New frontiers in the future of aging: from successful aging of the young old to the dilemmas of the fourth age. *Gerontology* **49**: 123–135.

Berg, C.A., Upchurch, R. (2007) A developmental–contextual model of couples coping with chronic illness across the adult life span. *Psychological Bulletin* **133**(6): 920–954.

Bronfenbrenner, U. (1986) Ecology of the family as the context for human development. *Developmental Psychology* **22**: 723–742.

Bronfenbrenner, U. (1989) Ecological systems theory. *Annals of child development* **6**: 187–249.

Cairns, R.B., Elder, G.H., Costello, E.J. (eds) (1996) *Developmental Science.* Cambridge University Press: New York.

Carstensen, L.L. (2006) The influence of a sense of time on human development. *Science* **312**: 1913–1915.

Carstensen, L.L., Fung, H.H., Charles, S.T. (2003) Socioemotional selectivity theory and the regulation of emotion in the second half of life. *Motivation and Emotion* **27**(2): 103–123.

Christian, B. (2003) Growing up with chronic illness: psychosocial adjustment of children and adolescents with cystic fibrosis. *Annual Review of Nursing Research* **21**: 151–172.

Christian, B.J., D'Auria, J. (2006) Building life skills for children with cystic fibrosis. Effectiveness of an intervention. *Nursing Research* **55**(5): 300–307.

Christian, B.J., D'Auria, J., Moore, C.B. (1999) Playing for time: adolescent perspectives of lung transplantation for cystic fibrosis. *Journal of Pediatric Health Care* **13**: 120–125.

Cystic Fibrosis Foundation (CFF). (2004) *Cystic Fibrosis Foundation National CF Patient Registry: Annual Report 2003.* Cystic Fibrosis Foundation: Bethesda, MD.

Damon, W., Hart, D. (1992) Self-understanding and its role in social and moral development. In: Bornstein, M.H., Lamb, M.E. (eds) *Developmental Psychology: An Advanced Textbook*, 3rd edition. Erlbaum: Hillsdale, NJ, pp. 421–464.

Ebner, N., Freund, A.M., Baltes, P.B. (2006) Developmental changes in personal goal orientation from young to late adulthood: from striving for gains to maintenance and prevention of losses. *Psychology and Aging* **21**(4): 664–678.

Ekman, S.L., Norberg, A., Wahlin, T.B., Winblad, B. (1995) Dimensions and progression in the interaction between bilingual/monolingual caregivers and bilingual demented immigrants: analysis of video-recorded morning care sessions in institutions coded by means of the Erikson theory of 'eight stages of man'. *International Journal of Aging and Human Development* **41**(1): 29–45.

Erikson, E.H. (1964) *Insight and Responsibility*. Norton & Company: New York.

Erikson, E.H. (1982) *The Life Cycle Completed*. Norton & Company: New York.

Erikson, E.H., Erikson, J.M. (1981) On generativity and identity. *Harvard Educational Review* **51**: 249–269.

Erikson, E.H., Erikson, J.M., Kivnick, H.O. (1986) *Vital Involvement in Old Age*. Norton & Company: New York.

Gluckman, P.D., Hanson, M.A., Beedle, A.S. (2007) Early life events and their consequences for later disease: a life history and evolutionary perspective. *American Journal of Human Biology* **19**: 1–19.

Goodman, J., Schlossberg, N.K., Anderson, M.L. (2006) *Counselling Adults in Transition. Linking Practice with Theory*, 3rd edition. Springer: New York.

Hallberg, I.R. (1990) *Vocally disruptive behaviour in severely demented patients in relation to institutional care provided*. Umeå University Medical Dissertations, Sweden.

Kihlgren, M. (1992) *Integrity promoting care of demented patients*. Umeå University Medical Dissertations, Sweden.

Kihlgren, M., Hallgren, A., Norberg, A., Karlson, I. (1996) Disclosure of basic strengths and basic weaknesses in demented patients during morning care, before and after staff training: analysis of video-recordings by means of the Erikson theory of 'eight stages of man'. *International Journal of Aging and Human Development* **43**(3): 219–233.

Kihlgren, M., Kuremyr, D., Norberg, A. *et al.* (1993) Nurse-patient interaction after training in integrity promoting care at a long-term ward: analysis of videorecorded morning care sessions. *International Journal of Nursing Studies* **30**(1): 1–13.

Kirkevold, M. (2002) The unfolding illness trajectory of stroke. *Disability and Rehabilitation* **24**(17): 887–898.

Kleinman, A. (1988) *The Illness Narratives: Suffering, Healing, and the Human Condition*. Basic Books: New York.

Kvigne, K., Kirkevold, M., Gjengedal, E. (2005) The nature of nursing care and rehabilitation of female stroke survivors: the perspective of hospital nurses. *Journal of Clinical Nursing* **14**(7): 897–905.

Löckenhoff, C.E., Carstensen, L.L. (2007) Aging, emotion, and health-related decision strategies: motivational manipulations can reduce age differences. *Psychology and Aging* **22**(1): 134–146.

Macdonald, K. (2006) Living in limbo – patients with cystic fibrosis waiting for transplant. *British Journal of Nursing* **15**(10): 566–572.

Mamhidir, A.G., Karlsson, I., Norberg, A., Kihlgren, M. (2007) Weight increase in patients with dementia, and alternation in meal routines and meal environments after integrity promoting care. *Journal of Clinical Nursing* **16**: 987–996.

Miles, M.S., Holditch-Davis, D. (2003) Enhancing nursing research with children and families using a developmental science perspective. *Annual Review of Nursing Research* **21**: 1–20.

Norberg, A., Sandman, P.O. (1988) Existential dimensions of eating in Alzheimer's patients. An analysis by means of E.H. Erikson's theory of 'eight stages of man'. *Recent Advances in Nursing Science* **21**: 127–134.

Paterson, B.L. (2001) The shifting perspectives model of chronic illness. *Journal of Nursing Scholarship* **33**(1): 21–26.

Piaget, J. (2002) Judgment and reasoning in the child. International library of psychology. *Developmental Psychology*, Vol. 23. Routledge: London.

Putnam, M. (2002) Linking aging theory and disability models: increasing the potential to explore aging with physical impairment. *Gerontologist* **42**(6): 799–806.

Rankin, S.H., Weekes, D.P. (1989) Life-span development: a review of theory and practice for families with chronically ill members. *Scholarly Inquiry for Nursing Practice* **3**(1): 3–22.

Rankin, S.H., Weekes, D.P. (2000) Life-span development: a review of theory and practice for families with chronically ill members. *Scholarly Inquiry for Nursing Practice* **14**(4): 355–373.

Rolland, J.S. (1987) Chronic illness and the life cycle: a conceptual framework. *Family Process* **26**: 203–221.

Schlossberg, N.L. (1981) A model for analyzing human adaptation to transition. *The Counselling Psychologist* **9**: 2–18.

Smith, G.D. (2007) Life-course approaches to inequalities in adult chronic disease risk. *Proceedings of the Nutrition Society* **66**: 216–236.

Sroufe, L.A., Cooper, R.G., DeHart, G.B. (1996) *Child Development: Its Nature and Course*, 3rd edition. McGraw-Hill: New York.

Weekes, D.P. (1995) Adolescents growing up chronically ill: a life-span developmental view. *Family and Community Health* **17**(4): 22–34.

4. *Assisting People with Chronic Illness to Manage Co-Morbid Conditions*

Allison Williams

Introduction

The purpose of this chapter is to provide an overview of how co-morbidity has been conceptualised within the various health-care disciplines which have contributed to the fragmentation, replication and omissions in the care of people with co-morbidities. The specialisation of medicine, the way mental and physical health are viewed separately and the divisions in systems of care delivery add to the difficulties in managing co-morbidities and viewing the person with multiple chronic problems as a whole. The inequities in health care and the influences of the social determinants of how people with co-morbidity respond to and manage their health is also discussed. The debate about how best to manage multiple chronic illnesses from the viewpoint of various stakeholders is highlighted, drawing attention to the need for longitudinal approaches to health-care delivery to ensure the continuity of care. Emerging trends and innovative interventions that help people with co-morbidities and their family/significant others to transcend care frameworks offer promise for the future. Areas of research that are of a high priority are detailed throughout.

Complex behavioural change is necessary to manage the various treatments and follow-up that co-morbidities demand. A number of theoretical models to enable behaviour change in chronic illness exist (Dunbar-Jacob 2007). For example, the modified Health Belief Model (Murray-Johnson *et al.* 2000; Glanz *et al.* 2002) explains long-term health behaviours by focusing on the attitudes and beliefs of individuals and their perceived threat and net benefits of taking positive health-related action. However, this model has a Western capitalist focus and a narrow view of how people choose to live with chronic illness. Other models, such as the biopsychosocial model, are experiencing a revival in the social sciences. Nearly all models contain a component of education and self-efficacy – the confidence to carry out behaviours necessary to reach a goal identified by the consumer

(Bodenheimer *et al.* 2002). However, these theoretical models are not specifically designed for the complex interplay of co-morbidities that cross specialties, and alternatives to entrenched conceptual models designed for the recipients of Western health-care services would be an innovation in chronic illness research.

Conceptualising co-morbidity

Irrespective of the epidemiology, chronic illnesses are an escalating global health-care problem and are, by their definition, incurable; the more chronic illnesses the person has, the more complex are the treatment regimens and the impact on usual activities of daily living (Lubkin & Larsen 2002; Bayliss *et al.* 2007). *Chronic illness* is defined as 'a permanently altered health state, caused by a non-reversible pathological condition that leaves residual disability that cannot be corrected by a simple surgical procedure or cured by a short course of medical therapy' (Miller 1992, p. 4). Co-morbidities refer to two or more chronic illnesses in a person at the same time that are not directly related to the primary diagnosis (Nardi *et al.* 2007). People with co-morbidities require long-term health maintenance and self-management that includes frequent visits to health practitioners, interventions to control symptoms and disease progression and the management of personal emotions and family upheaval. Additionally, as chronic illnesses deteriorate over time, the severity of symptoms such as fatigue and pain increases, limiting the people's ability to live independently and manage their illnesses.

While co-morbidity has been broadly defined in the literature, the term has many meanings. One of the earliest medical definitions of co-morbidity used to research the possible influence of co-morbidities on the outcomes of diabetes was described as 'any distinct additional clinical entity' (Feinstein 1970, p. 456). Other researchers have defined co-morbidity as a medical problem not related to the primary diagnosis, another chronic condition, co-occurring psychopathology, inclusive of acute conditions, a complication and a combination of acute and chronic illnesses (Williams & Botti 2002). Such 'non-disease' entities as pregnancy or 'curable' problems such as tinea, dental problems, nosocomial infections and pressure ulcers were referred to as co-morbidities, whereas cancer was excluded. Brailer *et al.* (1996) attempted to carefully differentiate between the diagnosis at admission, secondary diagnosis, complication and co-morbidity but failed to clarify whether co-morbidities were strictly chronic in nature. Inconsistent definitions of co-morbidity reflect the needs of various players in health care which make it difficult to fully understand the implications of co-morbidities, much less to apply research findings to practice.

A further issue concerning the lack of a clear definition of co-morbidities relates to the way co-morbidities are recorded in various studies. For example, some researchers count co-morbidities present on admission to hospital but exclude complications that occur as a result of the admission, which might be included in other studies (Williams & Botti 2002). Studies have used consumer self-report for collecting data, which may not always be accurate. The consumer's willingness to disclose illnesses may be influenced by the stigma associated with particular co-morbidities and whether the illness is physically visible or not (Joachim & Acorn 2000). Other studies employ medical records that under-record co-morbidities, or administrative data sets that often limit the number of conditions that can be listed (de Groot *et al.* 2003; Lee *et al.* 2005).

The ability to estimate accurate prevalence rates is compounded by the fact that chronic illnesses have no clear onset or end to them (Gignac & Cott 1998). Thus, it is not clear from the medical literature what co-morbidity actually is, or how to accurately determine how many co-morbidities are present or their severity. Hence, co-morbidities have been conceptualised as an added burden that complicates the interest under study and, as such, are seen to be a major problem. As a result, co-morbidities are not appropriately recognised which makes the care of people with co-morbidities difficult to achieve. Failure to accurately record co-morbidities in clinical notes has implications for health professionals guided by these notes when they attempt to provide comprehensive care.

The prevalence of chronic illnesses is similar among developed countries, and research indicates that illnesses are most obvious when they affect an individual's everyday life and physical functioning rather than their mortality risk. Prevalence studies drawn from medical records, the *International Classification of Diseases Ninth Revision* (ICD-9) lexicon and national surveys reflect a medical interest in individual diseases for the purposes of clear diagnostic criteria, treatment guidelines and estimation of mortality risk rather than the provision of long-term care (Verbrugge & Patrick 1995). Although the *International Classification of Diseases Tenth Revision* (ICD-10) included the addition of ambulatory and managed care, it is primarily the collection, processing, classification and presentation of mortality statistics.

The recording of illness severity is another issue in co-morbidity management (Chan *et al.* 1997; de Groot *et al.* 2003). A systematic review of the validity and reliability of various methods of measuring the severity of co-morbidity has been conducted (de Groot *et al.* 2003). Four methods were identified as valid and reliable measures in clinical research from the health professional's perspective: the Cumulative Illness Rating Scale, the Charlson Index, the Index of Coexisting Disease and the Kaplan Index (de Groot *et al.* 2003). However, the Charlson Index was developed to predict patient mortality, the Kaplan Index was specifically designed for patients with diabetes and the Index of Coexisting Disease was developed to measure the disease severity in the context of the disability. The Cumulative Illness Rating Scale is the only instrument currently available that measures the burden and disease stability of physical and somatic co-morbidities according to body systems (Linn *et al.* 1968; Miller *et al.* 1992; Nardi *et al.* 2007). Other tools such as the APACHE 11 uses acute physiological parameters, age and pre-existing co-morbidities, to predict patient mortality in acute care settings, in particular, critical care which is not useful for persons with co-morbidities living in the community.

The severity of the illness plays an important role in people's perceptions of their quality of life and long-term health behaviours. Quality of life issues become increasingly important as the population ages. Quality of life is a multidimensional and subjective concept and generally refers to physical and mental well-being from the consumer's point of view (Schirm 2002). The person's functional capacity to carry out activities of daily living is an important indicator of his or her quality of life and is dependent on the type of illness, the overall disease burden and how the person adapts to his or her illness (Laukkanen *et al*. 1997). Quality of life is not easily addressed or measured, although numerous measures of general well-being and quality of life claim to explore the consumer's perspective (Garratt *et al*. 2002; Hawthorne & Osbourne 2005).

Co-morbidities affect quality of life, yet few researchers have studied the impact on quality of life (Fortin *et al*. 2002; Bayliss *et al*. 2007). It is assumed that co-morbidities negatively affect quality of life. Certainly, research demonstrates that coexisting musculoskeletal conditions and the renal system, which commonly involves co-morbidities and significant discomfort, have the most significant negative effects on quality of life (Kempen *et al*. 1997; Picavet & Hoeymans 2004). Chronic pain may be much more than a detriment to quality of life as research has shown that medical co-morbidity was a strong discriminator of subjects with chronic low back pain and those who were pain free; this requires further investigation (Rudy *et al*. 2007).

Options to improve quality of life become increasingly complex as the number of illnesses increase and may result in better illness management but no improvement in the quality of life. The social construction of co-morbidities has resulted in people being perceived to be 'too hard' to take care of and the perception that 'nothing helps'. Consumers often turn to complementary therapies in an attempt to control symptoms and although researchers report their effectiveness (Vas *et al*. 2004), there are very few clinical trials supporting their use.

Health professionals are challenged to identify effective ways to promote health, provide comfort and support the well-being of consumers with co-morbidities to maximise their self-efficacy. Trajectories have been developed in an attempt to describe the similarities and differences of chronic illnesses from a social rather than a biomedical perspective (Rolland 1987; Corbin & Strauss 1991). Morse (1997), Paterson (2001) and Kralik (2002) have challenged linear trajectories of chronic illness by emphasising that living with chronicity is a continually changing process. Once one illness becomes unstable, other co-morbidities recede into the background and are not as significant at that particular period in the person's life (Williams 2004).

The World Health Organization International Classification of Impairment, Disability and Handicap 2 (ICIDH 2) is a rehabilitation model that adopted an 'illness consequence' focus rather than a 'diagnosis and treat' acute disease focus of the first ICIDH model (Burton 2000). However, an unforeseen consequence of this model is the emphasis on the 'sick role' and the burden of disease that is value laden (Pfeiffer 2000), creating a bleak picture for the individual and family trying to maximise the rest of the life left to live.

Social determinants of co-morbidities

Socio-demographic influences on health are significant where disadvantaged groups are more likely to have poorer health and particular client groups such as the poor, mentally ill, ethnic and cultural minority groups and those from rural regions are at risk of inequitable care (Lubkin & Larsen 2002). In addition, the ageing population and a change in the social structure mean people more often live alone and are in need of formal or informal help that the health system is not always able to provide (Temmink *et al.* 2000). This situation undermines a person's ability to take positive health actions. It is apparent that the health-care systems of Western countries are barely sustainable and will only become further burdened by the increasing prevalence of co-morbidities (Saltman 2005). Health systems need to tailor care models to cope with their increased prevalence, requiring a radical revisioning of chronic illness management beyond prescribed medications.

Some changes in prevalence reflect evolving medical and social influences in public health. Diabetes is becoming increasingly widespread (Gross *et al.* 2005) and up to 40% of consumers with diabetes will also develop kidney disease (Thomas & Atkins 2006). Whatever their epidemiology, co-morbidities increase the risk of dependency and the need for care where daily decisions need to be made by the persons living independently in the community regarding their treatment options and follow-up. As a result of the poor outcomes of diabetes, authorities are recommending strong preventative measures and increasingly vigilant strategies to ensure early diagnosis and management in an attempt to prevent further illness and reduce associated health-care costs (Colman *et al.* 1999). Expert consumers with co-morbidities need supportive health professionals from a wide range of disciplines and health-care agencies to facilitate self-management within a collaborative economic, social and political health-care system to maintain well-being and prevent further illness.

The medical paradigm

The management of Western health-care systems is clearly influenced by the dominance of the biomedical approach of diagnosis, cause and cure, which is not appropriate for chronic conditions. The use of the term disease rather than illness or chronic condition reflects the medical framework used to treat the problem, rather than learning to adapt and live with it (Lubkin & Larsen 2002). The construction of chronic illness is rooted in medical discourses of science, normalisation and individualism, which has not facilitated the appropriate care of the person with chronic illnesses (Wellard 1998). Lifestyle aspects such as obesity, lack of regular exercise, nutritional inadequacies, smoking, certain occupations and previous trauma play a significant role in the development of illness (Dunstan *et al.* 2002; Powell *et al.* 2005). While scientific breakthroughs offer cures at the microscopic level, the social influences on health and illness are important in the long haul of established illness management.

Until chronic diseases can be cured, health professionals using the medical model can become frustrated with increasingly complex treatments and exhausted treatment options. Under the medical model, people with co-morbidities have been subjected to unnecessary diagnostic and therapeutic interventions to predict the effectiveness of uncertain treatments (Rutledge *et al.* 2001). The diagnostic focus of health care is demonstrated by Australian statistics showing that a third of admissions to public hospitals in 2002–2003 were for investigative procedures (Australian Institute of Health & Welfare 2004). Once diagnoses are confirmed, the incurable nature of chronic diseases means that medical treatment has a limited effectiveness in controlling symptoms and disease progression (Foster *et al.* 2003). These issues are compounded in the presence of co-morbidities (Redelmeier *et al.* 1998).

Since Verbrugge *et al.*'s groundbreaking study (1989), much of the scientific research on co-morbidity continues to address classification systems of co-morbidities, the consequences of having co-morbidities in the context of disability, mental illness, institutionalisation, death, frequencies in populations, economic consequences and, to a lesser extent, the theories about disease co-occurrence. In addition, various medical co-morbidity indices have been developed to predict mortality risk, surgical complication rates, resource utilisation and treatment evaluation, rather than the person's overall functional ability and quality of life (Williams & Botti 2002). Research often excludes patients with co-morbidities in order to increase trial efficiency and the ability to generalise the findings (de Groot *et al.* 2003). Additionally, researching idiosyncratically occurring co-morbidities makes scientific rigour and sampling of particular co-morbid conditions difficult to achieve.

Functional impairments, physical discomfort and psychosocial changes such as changes in lifestyle, role changes, identity transformations and spiritual crises demonstrate that living with a chronic illness is enmeshed in everyday life where the medical model seems irrelevant. Psychosocial interventions to enable long-term behavioural change in Western models of health care are yet to be fully examined, in addition to exploring different adaptive models to illness.

Medical research is tackling related pairs of chronic conditions such as hyperlipidemia and diabetes (Parris *et al.* 2005), hyperlipidemia and heart disease (Bouchard *et al.* 2007), obesity and heart disease (Gregg *et al.* 2005) and obesity and osteoarthritis (Dunlop *et al.* 2005). Synergistic effects of combinations of particular diseases have been reported (Verbrugge *et al.* 1989; Rijken *et al.* 2005). However, very few studies have investigated the relationship of multiple combinations of chronic illnesses (Walker 2005), reflecting the damaging reputation of co-morbidities.

Most researchers reported co-morbidity in the title of their studies, which were in the context of mental health and combinations of medical and psychiatric illness research were uncommon, reflecting the Cartesian mind–body split. This was a surprising finding, as people with a mental illness have a similar prevalence of physical illnesses as the general population (McCormick *et al.* 1994); in some cases, people with mental illness have a higher prevalence of common chronic conditions such as osteoporosis, cardiovascular disease and diabetes than the general population (Leucht *et al.* 2007). Additionally, the development of a secondary somatic chronic illness is commonly associated with subsequent depression (Sprangers *et al.* 2000; Lapsley *et al.* 2001). Good mental health is necessary to facilitate coping, resilience and learning new skills and information needed to manage physical co-morbidities in the long term.

Dual diagnosis is almost exclusively in the domain of psychiatry where a plethora of studies investigating combinations of mental illness and substance abuse exists. These 'double trouble' illnesses often exacerbate each other and have overlapping symptoms making treatment especially difficult. However, in Canada, dual diagnosis may refer to an individual with both a mental illness and a developmental disability. Whatever the case, dual diagnosis rarely encapsulates medical and mental conditions together unless it concerns the consequences of substance abuse and risk-taking behaviour such as illicit drug use and HIV.

The prevalence of mental health dual diagnosis is increasing. However, treatment is fragmented by a lack of integration within the speciality. Consumers with dual diagnosis may receive treatment in either a mental health facility or a detoxification unit, placing them at an increased risk of physical illness, social isolation and self-harm (Nader 2007). Similarly, consumers with mental health problems who require acute care services for a physical illness are at risk of inadequate care of their mental illness during their hospital stay (de Crespigny *et al.* 2002). The socio-political implications of combining illnesses that have received negative press have important ramifications for the future development of integrated health-care approaches. Integration of mental health and drug services has begun in some countries, although staffing profiles are significantly different for each subspecialty, which complicate their integration (DHS 2007).

Interest in concomitant mental and physical or surgical diagnoses remains uncommon and researchers tend to confine co-morbidities to their respective body system or sub-system of interest. Exceptions included studies that investigated ageing processes such as dementia and heart failure (McGann 2000) and diabetes and depression (Kalsekar *et al.* 2006). In addition, the prevalence of consumers with both physical and mental illnesses has been obscured by current data collection methods. For example, mental illnesses have been recorded separately from physical chronic illnesses in national health databases. Therefore, people suffering a combination of somatic and mental chronic illnesses are more difficult to locate and may not be easily included in research (Sprangers *et al.* 2000; Saltman 2005).

The division between mental and physical health and the increasing specialisation of health care to the extent of sub-specialisations within body systems has particular implications for people suffering from co-morbidities, given that specialisation is likely to fragment treatment by focusing on individual illnesses (Smith & O'Dowd 2007). To illustrate this point, there are currently more than 2000 categories of health professionals in the United States, compared with 10 categories 50 years ago (Lawrence 2002). A similar trend is observed in Australia, with currently more than 75 areas of defined nursing practice. It is evident that a comprehensive, multidisciplinary approach to managing chronic illnesses with quality communication, supports and referral processes is needed in order to deliver a coordinated continuity of care (Williams 2004).

The prevention and management of co-morbidities require a sustained, complex behavioural change where adherence is a significant problem. Different diets, medications and self-monitoring, disease management advocated by various specialists and an interdisciplinary team are required by the expert consumer to cope. Adherence, compliance and, more recently, concordance have been used interchangeably in the literature; although adherence involves consumer choice and is intended to be non-judgmental, compliance reflects a biomedical paradigm that reinforces patient passivity, and concordance refers to a consultative partnership between the consumer and health professional (Roter *et al.* 1998; WHO 2003; Haynes *et al.* 2005).

The medical model's chief treatment of chronic disease is prescribed medications. It is generally accepted that the effectiveness of medications and their long-term outcomes depend on the person's adherence to the prescribed regimen on a regular basis (WHO 2003). However, safe and effective medicine management has traditionally been examined according to the biomedical characteristics of medicines, such as the complexity of dosage, method of administration, frequency of use, side effects and how they affect body processes (Galbraith *et al.* 2007). The reliance on pharmacology when faced with the problem of co-morbidities overlooks alternative strategies that may be more helpful and less intrusive to the consumer, particularly in the case of depression that often accompanies chronic somatic illnesses (Gask 2005b).

When different body systems are diseased, there may be diametrically opposed treatment strategies that result in the treatment of one disease being prioritised over that of another, creating physiological challenges and conflicting information for the consumer. For example, second-generation antipsychotics used to treat schizophrenia can cause severe weight gain, which, in the presence of cardiovascular disease or diabetes, complicates management. The treatment of osteoarthritis with nonsteroidal anti-inflammatory drugs (NSAIDs) is contraindicated in chronic kidney disease and people with multiple sclerosis are advised to rest, whereas if they also have osteoarthritis, movement and exercise are advocated. Attempting to adhere to multiple treatments based on single diseases can be harmful (Bayliss *et al.* 2007).

This situation is made more complicated when the illness is asymptomatic and the consumer cannot feel the benefit of taking the medication (Vermeire *et al.* 2005). In addition, most pharmacokinetic studies of prescribed medicines designed to halt disease progression assume medication adherence, leading to concerns about the validity of the findings. Studies are needed to clarify the benefits of medication adherence on health outcomes as people can improve or deteriorate for reasons other than taking medicines as prescribed (Vermeire *et al.* 2005; Lindenmeyer *et al.* 2006; Schroeder *et al.* 2006).

Johnson *et al.* (2005) examined risk factors for untoward medication events in older people and found that taking more than 12 medicines per day, having more than one prescriber, the presence of a caregiver and forgetfulness were related to adherence, providing risk factors for screening clients for potential medicine-related problems.

Polypharmacy and complementary therapies in people with chronic illnesses highlight concerns about medicine-related adverse events and the safety and benefits of complementary therapies, which has been extensively reported in the literature in the context of single chronic conditions (Grant *et al.* 2003; Zochling *et al.* 2004), but rarely in the context of co-morbidities.

While side effects are a particular concern for people taking multiple medications, adhering to prescribed regimens for a long term may be more problematic for the consumer. Adherence is the extent to which the person continues taking medicines as prescribed under limited supervision when faced with conflicting demands and it has most commonly been assessed by determining how well consumers follow health-related advice and prescription refills rather than by exploring how lifestyle and socio-environmental factors affect the individual's ability to adhere (Alexander *et al.* 2003).

A number of studies have assessed the interventions for improving adherence in particular medical conditions or monotherapies, but few have significantly affected clinical outcomes (Haynes *et al.* 2005; Kripalani *et al.* 2007). Research focusing on the medicinal concerns of individuals with a single chronic illness simplifies the intricacy of health issues of people with multiple health problems. Little information is available regarding the reasons as to why people stop treatment. Pound *et al.* (2005) analysed the qualitative studies of why people resist taking medicines, reporting that people do not adhere to their prescribed medicine regimens primarily because of concerns about the side effects of medicines rather than forgetfulness, as found by other studies using quantitative methodologies.

Interactive instructional interventions to aid decision-making offer innovative approaches to assist consumers with diverse backgrounds and Internet access to understand their illnesses and complex medication regimens (Murray *et al.* 2005). Additionally, cost-effective electronic health care delivered over the Internet offers a major potential in helping people to manage their co-morbidities independently (Duke 2005). The possibility of disseminating key health messages to remote populations with access to technology is a significant development in chronic illness management.

Health-care systems

Health-care systems are changing to better meet the needs of chronic illness as chronic illnesses by far represent the largest disease burden in Western countries. However, the current health system was designed to meet acute care needs rather than the needs of an ageing chronically ill society (Rothman & Wagner 2003; Nardi *et al.* 2007). Patients in acute hospital medical wards are mostly older and have multiple co-morbid conditions that require complex and holistic care that the systems of casemix, diagnosis related groups (DRGs) and administrative management systems do little to promote (Williams & Botti 2002; Nardi *et al.* 2007). In effect, health-care planners have not been very visionary in predicting the needs of people with chronic illnesses. Health services are demand driven, fee-for-service and fragmented at local and national levels around the globe. The imbalance in the provision of health care has risked a shift from needs assessment to economic rationing (Parry-Jones & Soulsby 2001). Suggestions that clinical governance provides a new process model to drive quality of care (Nardi *et al.*

2007) has been met with some scepticism in the workplace because it closely resembles previous risk management programmes and as such lacks innovation.

Different chronic conditions have different outcomes and conditions that have a large impact on the population may not be given the same funding as those that have negative outcomes (Badley & Glazier 2004). Non-fatal chronic conditions far outweigh fatal diseases and receive a disproportionate use of health services (Verbrugge & Patrick 1995; Lubkin & Larsen 2002; Badley & Glazier 2004). For example, hypertension has been labelled the 'silent killer' and is more likely to attract funding rather than non-fatal arthritis and chronic back pain, which incur major functional impairment on a daily basis. Urinary incontinence, which is associated with many co-morbid conditions, imposes a significant burden on the person and health-care resources (Doran *et al.* 2001; Hu *et al.* 2004). Health professionals working in partnership with consumers can enhance their self-efficacy and expert skills in managing urinary incontinence independently to improve control over their life and its quality (Kralik *et al.* 2007).

The frequent user of health-care services, the person with co-morbidities, has to navigate a complex health-care system to receive the care they consider appropriate. Casemix, diagnosis-related groups and clinical pathways have been introduced into the acute care sector to deliver health services in the shortest possible time frame and at the least cost. Despite widespread efforts to standardise health-care utilisation in Western countries, there are significant differences in the length of stay for comparable chronic illnesses between institutions and countries. The variability is attributed in part to variations in medical practices and the type and availability of support after discharge (Cleary *et al.* 1991). Research that reduced lengths of stay and changes in methods of payment for health care in an attempt to contain health-care costs have resulted in poor continuity of care, unplanned hospital readmission and cost shifting (Anderson *et al.* 2005). Uninsured older people with co-morbidities have been found to deteriorate more rapidly under public health care when compared to those who have health insurance (Ware *et al.* 1996; Raddish *et al.* 1999). Therefore, people most likely to suffer from failures in the health-care system are those who need it the most.

Effective chronic illness management requires more than adding to a system focused on acute care; it requires attention to the design of the delivery system (Wagner *et al.* 2002). Western health-care systems are not designed to reimburse the type of supportive care people with chronic illnesses need. Health systems can promote continuity of care by valuing it through the provision of adequate resources, time and systems that facilitate assessment, appropriate referral systems, communication and planning. Recognition of a multidisciplinary approach in partnership with the consumer is needed to provide quality of care and to enhance health outcomes.

In the workplace, the quality of a patient's assessment is critical. However, a lack of time often prevents illnesses secondary to the presenting problem from being assessed during consultations, where a supportive health-care system recognises and values the additional time that chronic illness management entails. Longer consultation times need to be used productively, to allow the consumer to express their concerns freely and not be dominated by experts

(Rycroft-Malone *et al.* 2001; Stevenson *et al.* 2004). A collaborative relationship between the doctor and patient facilitates emergence of the 'expert patient' to self-manage co-morbidities independently (Paterson *et al.* 2001). Health-care reforms that demand more complex care delivery in shorter time frames increase work-load and have been linked to job dissatisfaction, burnout and concerns about the quality of care (Aiken *et al.* 2002). These issues are compounded by the complexity of care spawned by co-morbidities (Redelmeier *et al.* 1998).

Significant health-care reforms are underway in Western countries with the implementation of new policies and programmes to lessen the growing burden of chronic illness. Innovative programmes include the UK Expert Patients Programme of primary health-care reform involving self-management initiatives (Kennedy *et al.* 2007). Private health-care companies in the United States have claimed implementing 'one-stop shops' for a broad range of post-acute services for their paying members to overcome fragmentation of services. In the public health-care system, programmes have been established to enable support of patients in their home by hospital staff after discharge from acute care (Sparbel & Anderson 2000). However, these initiatives require appropriate resources and research to ensure optimal patient outcomes, and the consumer's perspective in shaping health-care services has not been well conveyed (Poulton 1999).

Other strategies to reduce the cost of managing chronic illness include the emerging 'substitution of care' initiative in Australia, Canada, Europe and the United States where unqualified staff are employed at the lowest cost to care for people with chronic illnesses (Temmink *et al.* 2000; Stone 2004). The trend for employing unregulated staff in aged care is a specific concern, particularly given that these people are expected to provide care at the very time it is at its most complex (Nay *et al.* 1999). The self-managing consumer with co-morbidities who is not reimbursed for his or her out-of-pocket health-care expenses is also a cheaper alternative for governments trying to contain health-care costs.

People with co-morbidities frequently experience personal economic pressures in addition to the health problems incurred because of their illnesses that include the loss of employment and paying additional health costs. Medical under-treatment of consumers' co-morbidities may be more common when the treatment involves out-of-pocket expenses not covered by health-care plans (Steinbrook 1998; Lapsley *et al.* 2001; Alexander *et al.* 2003). Families absorb health-care costs which often means that they have to make sacrifices in other areas such as social, nutritional and lifestyle activities which may not always be healthy choices.

The increasing cost shifting towards the family in providing care in the face of limited external support raises major issues for health workers concerned with the people's welfare and equitable health care (Parker 1999). Carers are often older and have chronic illnesses and can become overwhelmed with increasingly complex treatment and care and may sacrifice their own medical care in the process (MacLennan 1998). The resultant caregiver burden can lead to the consumer having unmet needs or being institutionalised prematurely.

There is minimal evidence of literature or experience of co-morbidity outside of developed countries. The cultural and physiological aspects of the co-morbidity experience affect how people live with chronic illness. For instance, netting is emphasised as a way of preventing malaria in Africa, but antimalarial medications are much less common, resulting in disease prevention without meaningful follow-through for many Africans. This situation affects the development and experience of chronic illnesses in general and perpetuates myths that are counterproductive to health. As screening is not routine and health care depends on available funding, many diseases remain undiagnosed until the damage reaches the end stage, as in kidney disease, diabetes, hypertension and HIV (Naicker 2003). Similarly, Asian countries have a high incidence of tuberculosis, diabetes and HIV with inequitable access to medications compared to Western countries: more than one-third of the global population does not have equitable access to essential medicines proven to reduce mortality and morbidity (Cohen-Kohler 2007).

Co-morbidity management

The acute care setting

In the acute care setting, contemporary specialised medical care is capable of repairing many acute medical problems after which patients can usually return to their previous autonomous lives, free from disease. This is not the case for people with co-morbidities. In addition, when a patient with co-morbidities is admitted to an acute care setting, the staff focus on resolving the acute care problem. This is vital, so long as co-morbidities are not overlooked. However, short lengths of stay and clinical pathways that enhance the speciality focus of the acute admission do not lend themselves to co-morbidity care or the development of a trusting therapeutic relationship between the patient and members of the health-care team necessary for collaborative co-morbidity management (Williams *et al.* 2007).

There is minimal research relating to the management of people with co-morbidities in the acute care setting, the community or in transition between the hospital and community settings. People with co-morbidities have an increased symptom burden and are at risk of developing additional health problems which may discourage doctors from arranging surgical procedures for them (Levin *et al.* 2002). Studies have shown that co-morbidities such as surgery, complication rates, mortality, functional status, quality of life and hospital readmissions negatively influence the outcomes of hospital care and alter the course or outcome of the illnesses (Verbrugge *et al.* 1989; Williams & Botti 2002).

The effect of co-morbidities on surgical outcomes has not been well-addressed in past work, in particular joint replacement that is frequently performed in older people who have co-morbidities (McMurray *et al.* 2002; Williams *et al.* 2007). Previous research in joint replacement and co-morbidities has been limited by small sample sizes, patient populations from single institutions, inadequate control of variables and contradictory results (Keener *et al.* 2003; Jain *et al.* 2005). Long waiting lists for elective joint replacement surgery reflect the failings of the current health-care systems in meeting the needs of the chronically ill (Badley *et al.* 2007; Williams *et al.* 2007). Research strongly suggests that the total joint replacement conducted earlier in the course of a patient's functional decline may improve clinical outcomes (Fortin *et al.* 2002).

Discharge planning

Effective discharge planning relates to the health of the whole person, including health problems additional to the primary reason for admission, to ensure the seamless transition of the patient between the hospital and the community (Armitage & Kavanagh 1998). However, Papenhausen *et al.* (1998) claimed that health-care professionals in the hospital and community frequently pass the coordinating responsibilities for chronic illnesses back and forth which leads to duplicated and fragmented services, increased health-care costs and deteriorating health. Community nurses with inadequate resources also struggle to meet the needs of people with co-morbidities living at home. The continuity of care is especially problematic when the person is required to see and respond to a multitude of health professionals offering specialist advice and treatment.

Ideally, discharge planning commences when a patient prepares for an admission to acute care and is an interdisciplinary, hospital-wide process that helps patients and families develop feasible plans of care for after discharge; yet most research into discharge planning has not addressed all the phases of discharge planning or represented all the stakeholders (Hedges *et al.* 1999). Researchers have identified vulnerable groups of people such as older people who are discharged home 'quicker and sicker' in an attempt to contain health-care costs (Verbrugge *et al.* 1994; Williams & Botti 2002). Specific gaps in discharge planning have been identified that impact negatively on a person's quality of life post discharge; these gaps include delayed support systems and inadequate help from formal and informal providers (Armitage & Kavanagh 1998). Interestingly, wound management can be favourably implemented after discharge because such treatment fits well within the medical model of care and funding (Proctor *et al.* 1996).

Longitudinal studies into the post discharge needs of patients with co-morbidities is scarce, although Verbrugge *et al.* (1994) found that after a hospital stay, patients with co-morbidities had improved psychological functioning but their physical and social functioning lagged in comparison. In addition, fluctuation and decline in health status was noted up to 7–10 months post discharge. These periods of instability reinforce the need for long-term continuity of care for people with co-morbidities and the value of short reassessment intervals to measure true change when managing or conducting research about people with co-morbidities.

Models of chronic illness management

Diverse models of community care to meet the needs of people with chronic illnesses have been developed based on different types of health insurance and health-care policy. Although efforts are being made towards a longitudinal illness management model of care, current reimbursement models are disincentives for home-based care involving time-consuming care coordination, patient education and counselling (Long & Mann 1998; Bayliss *et al.* 2007), and contribute to doctors ignoring the presence of additional chronic conditions during consultation (Saltman 2005).

Chronic illness management tends to fall into three main models in order of increasing dependence on health-care self-management, disease management and case management. The value of the general practitioner (GP) over specialist care, multidisciplinary 'shared care', case management and disease management programmes in primary care have been reported (Rothman & Wagner 2003). Whichever model of chronic illness management is used, continuity of care is critical to reduce illness-related distress and serve as a gate-keeping function to facilitate access to other services (Ward 1990). The relationship between the health professional and consumer is critical in the provision of continuity of care. Continuity of care improves quality of care for consumers with chronic conditions, and this relationship has been consistently reported in the literature (Cabana & Jee 2004). Although continuity of care is seen to be defined as a series of connected patient-care events, both within a health-care institution and among multiple settings, it is multifactorial and poorly defined and reflects the stakeholders' motivation rather than the consumer's perspective (Sparbel & Anderson 2000; Haggerty *et al.* 2003).

Care of people with co-morbidities in general practice has been explored from the Australian perspective by Harris and Zwar (2007). As with the acute care system, specialists are unlikely to instigate treatment for diseases unrelated to their speciality, leaving general practice to be the key provider of continuity of care for co-morbidities. However, only about half of the patients receive optimal primary care. A variety of funding and chronic disease support infrastructure initiatives have been implemented that include practice nurse roles to help patients take on self-management skills. Nevertheless, administration burden, complex reimbursement methods and a lack of multidisciplinary teamwork, decision support systems and integration between the various stakeholders overseeing care remain obstacles to quality primary care of people with co-morbidities in Australia.

Self-management

Self-management programmes, the activities people undertake to manage their chronic illnesses and maintain their health, are proliferating as health-care workers endeavour to best meet the needs of consumers in the community (Lorig *et al.* 2004). Self-management programmes typically follow sociological approaches to help people in self-management of the medical aspects of their disease (drugs, diet and appointments), self-management of their role (job, family and friends) and emotional management in dealing with the illness on a daily basis (anger, fear, frustration and sadness). The positive and negative social influences affecting self-management requires investigation according to each illness and the type of support and self-management behaviour needed (Gallant 2003). Self-management needs to be individualised and needs to overcome difficulties at the patient, provider and health-care policy levels (Bayliss *et al.* 2007).

The management of chronic conditions depends on the person's illness behaviour which is influenced by access and perceived effectiveness of interventions to relieve symptoms, the type of intervention required, perceived illness severity, previous illness experiences, knowledge relating to the illness and psychosocial issues (Paterson 2001; Lubkin & Larsen 2002). Previous illness experiences shape the consumer's expectations, beliefs and self-management of the newly diagnosed disease. Paterson (2001) emphasises that living with chronicity is a continually changing process, where self-care varies and may at times seem neglectful, such as when taking drug holidays or during poor disease follow-up. People place different meanings on illness and have different perceptions that affect their self-care decision-making to enable them to cope with the reality of living with chronic conditions on a daily basis. A study conducted by Townsend *et al.* (2006), of participants negotiating four or more chronic illnesses, found that participants exhibited a moral obligation to manage 'well' and function socially despite experiencing discomfort: controlling symptoms was not always as rewarding as being able to live what they considered was a normal life and fulfil the usual roles.

Although people have similar generic self-care decisions that span chronic diseases, disease-specific perceptions influence these decisions that require consideration and exploration of why they are made (Paterson *et al.* 2002). Notions of self-care are especially important in people with co-morbidities who require multiple interventions and multidisciplinary management that requires an active expert consumer role, not the 'sick role' that paternalistic approaches foster. Adequate recognition and management of depressive symptoms that accompany co-morbidities that impede self-management is essential (Bayliss *et al.* 2007). Overarching, explicit principles of self-management are needed to transcend the various disciplines that are involved in facilitating the consumer to actively manage their illnesses.

Although Lorig *et al.* (1999, 2001) have reported successful generic self-management programmes that reduce health-care utilisation, the limitations of self-management programmes are prolific. Self-management programmes neglect the influence of co-morbidities, some chronic conditions do not respond well to self-management, they rely on the person's desire and ability to engage in self-management strategies and therefore may not target the people who need it most; they typically embrace a medical model of self-management focusing on taking prescribed medications, do not always reduce health-care expenditure and their efficacy over the long term has been questioned (Williams & Botti 2002). In addition, much effort is expended on a modest number of people to self-manage; for example, goal setting critical to self-management is time intensive, self-care skills training is not easily reimbursed, some people do not benefit from the group experience associated with self-management while others lack insight into how well they are actually self-managing. Health professionals' attitudes to self-management may also be a barrier (Blakeman *et al.* 2006) and would benefit from further research.

Self-management also favours a simplistic approach to health by reinforcing the 'successfully ill' and overplaying the success and enthusiasm of lay expertise that may not always be congruent with those of the health professional (Newbould *et al.* 2006). Self-management also neglects system failures in health care and different forms of non-biomedical influences and outcomes have yet to be explored. Additionally, self-management is difficult when health professionals do not adequately communicate with each other regarding a person's care, which increases the likelihood of duplicated services or incompatible treatments.

The research into chronic illness self-management research to date is difficult to analyse as it has been conducted without an agreed definition of what self-management means and has typically involved heterogeneous samples with different interventions, settings, personnel, programme formats and outcomes (Chodosh *et al.* 2005). In addition, the sustained behavioural change that self-management relies on has not been researched in studies beyond 2 years. Multidisciplinary disease management and disease self-management randomised controlled trials typically researched educational interventions for single illnesses such as heart disease and hypertension and used outcome measures of readmission, health-care utilisation or mortality, for example, Krumholz *et al.* (2002), Wright *et al.* (2003) and Figar *et al.* (2006). Health-care utilisation as an outcome may not be the most suitable measure, as health-care use is dynamic and dependent on the consumer's experience of his or her chronic illness and providers of health care (Gately *et al.* 2007). Importantly, the outcomes of self-management studies often do not include quality of life, which is the most important measure for the consumer living with chronic illnesses, in addition to out-of-pocket expenses. However, the study of Vale *et al.* (2003) on heart disease was unusual in that a coaching intervention improved quality of life and psychological health without attention to adherence. Another problem with self-management research is that chronic illnesses naturally progress over time and a significant number of participants will deteriorate despite good self-management.

Disease management

Cost containment and fragmented care have given rise to an escalation in disease management programmes to improve quality of life, health outcomes and patient satisfaction and to reduce health-care costs (Rothman & Wagner 2003; Krumholz *et al.* 2006). Disease management programmes are attempting to include patients with a wide range of co-morbidities to provide a more integrated approach to care (Krumholz *et al.* 2006). However, a lack of shared understanding of disease management programmes has constrained their evaluation, where a taxonomy has been developed to identify those who are most effective (Krumholz *et al.* 2006).

Disease management programmes have been challenged because the recommended interventions are often based on small data sets for a single chronic illness or patterns of interest (Kozma 1998). Disease management programmes also fail to fully conceptualise a consumer-centred process with collaborative partnerships between the consumer and health worker and affective strategies to assist disease management are not addressed (Krumholz *et al.* 2006). Disease management is complicated by research reporting that GPs do not always follow evidence-based guidelines (Sequist *et al.* 2005). However, physicians are not prepared adequately to care for the consumer with multiple chronic conditions and experience competing demands that require continual prioritising (Bayliss *et al.* 2007). Physicians' conformity to guidelines has been higher for patients with diabetes and hypertension than for patients with diabetes and kidney disease, demonstrating the complexity of managing diseases out of preferred specialties

(Cooke & Fatodu 2006). Certainly, longer appointment times with the GP would provide better chronic illness management in primary care (Campbell *et al.* 2001; Harris & Zwar 2007).

In chronic illness management, specialist knowledge needs to be more available to all health-care providers by developing linkages that cross practice and organisational boundaries to ensure that patients receive the best treatment (Gask 2005a). Additionally, quality primary care requires expert documentation and communication skills to enable the GP to make informed decisions. However, laboratory results, letters, X-ray results, history, physical examination and medication lists were not available in nearly 14% of primary care visits (Smith *et al.* 2005). The value of a consistent primary care provider is also not recognised by people who have multiple co-morbid conditions (Williams 2004). Electronic health records that provide a comprehensive overview of the consumer's care may overcome some of these barriers to continuity of care, but privacy issues impede their implementation, particularly in relation to the disclosure of mental illnesses.

Case management

Case management, the coordination of care across care areas, between agencies and their home, for complex patients and their families was developed as a means of ensuring quality care, cost-effectiveness and efficiency (Hovenga 1998; Schifalacqua *et al.* 2000). However, case management pathways often have been developed for single diagnoses, the disabled and the frail elderly rather than to assist the more common problem of consumers with complex co-morbidities. Likewise, the potential exists for competition and role confusion between case managers and other health providers and subsequent fragmentation of care (Sparbel & Anderson 2000).

The success of case management depends on the extent of programme integration with existing health-care services and any interagency collaborative effort, which is not always present (Alkema *et al.* 2003; Brand *et al.* 2004). Access to quality general practitioners and measures of continuity of care may be more reliable indicators of quality of care than readmission rates commonly reported in case management research (Brand *et al.* 2004; Aakvik & Holmas 2006). The long-term benefits of case management have yet to be captured (Gagnon *et al.* 1999). A common problem highlighted in the literature is the variability between standards of care of case managers in a system-centred rather than a client-centred service (Cooper & Yarmo Roberts 2006). Maintaining support for informal carers is also critical (MacLennan 1998).

Many randomised controlled trials have been conducted in an attempt to justify case management as a viable economic service in aged care, although substantial methodological challenges have made the analysis of research difficult (Brand *et al.* 2004). As reported by Diwan (1999) and Hadjistavropoulos *et al.* (2003), much of the literature on case management is descriptive and minimal empirical research has been conducted on the variables that influence case management services. Despite ambivalent results and reports that community-based, long-term care does not increase survival or affect deterioration in functional status, the demand for public community-based long-term programmes is strong and increasing (Kinney *et al.* 2003).

Little empirical research is available on the variables that contribute to a greater need for case management services, where client casemix within programmes may account for significant variations in cost (Diwan 1999; Hadjistavropoulos *et al.* 2003). The absence of details within studies describing the determinants of caseloads and caseload complexity undermines the capacity of the researchers to identify some of the causative factors that can support or hinder client and programme outcomes.

Case management is often applied in areas where the service delivery systems fail to meet the needs of 'complex' clients. Case managers practice within complex service systems, waiting lists, referral criteria, rules defining funding eligibility and expectations of quality on the part of service providers, consumers and funding bodies that add to the complexity of the client's situation. The allocation of the case management's resource seems to be determined by the capacity of case managers to meet the business needs of organisations offering case management. The absence of thorough investigation into the 'dosage' of case management is reflective of the challenges that surround workload measurement. This challenge should not deter researchers from examining more rigorously the effect that caseload and caseload complexity can have on client and programme outcomes, particularly where new technologies or novel approaches are being applied.

Conclusion

Co-morbidities have become an inevitable part of life for the vast majority of people. Interest in the overall problem of co-morbidities is increasing in response to their increasing prevalence and problems associated with their management. Research relating to co-morbidities has highlighted the fragmentation, replication and neglected care encountered when the person with co-morbidity is required to interact with a variety of practitioners in multiple health-care settings and an effort to self-manage complex treatments. In addition, the increasing specialisation in health care has particular implications for people suffering from co-morbidities, given that specialisation is likely to further fragment treatment by focusing on a particular illness. Models of chronic illness management and systems designed to integrate and coordinate chronic illness care are not designed for co-morbid conditions, and innovative models of co-morbidity management are needed.

The construction of co-morbidities has originated in medical discourses of curing, resulting in a perception that co-morbidities are dangerous, too hard to manage and are mostly associated with psychiatric conditions, contributing to stigma and less than optimal management. Given that the majority of Western society experiences a variety of somatic and psychiatric co-morbidities, a shift in the way chronic conditions are perceived is urgently required. In addition, a mandate to correct the disproportionate access the less fortunate have to health services is a moral and ethical obligation.

The practice implications for co-morbidity commence at the coalface and extend to the organisation of health care. Health-care professionals need to ask consumers about the impact of each co-morbidity on their lives and how best to meet their expectations. Consumers need to know about the key interactions that may occur between chronic conditions and prescribed medications and how to respond should these occur. The health-care consultation needs to be a partnership, where agreed treatment is negotiated between the provider and consumer: explorations of programmes that embrace concordance and operate from the consumer's lifeworld are essential. In the acute care setting, staff need to be cognizant of the additional care and treatment that co-morbidities require, including a thorough discharge plan and smooth transition back to the community. Quality communication among all members of the multidisciplinary team is essential.

Continuity of care is a major challenge in co-morbidity, and evidence-based interventions that assist people and their family/significant others to transcend care frameworks are critical. Longitudinal studies exploring psychosocial interventions that assist people to manage their co-morbidities represented a significant gap in the research. The use of information technology offers novel approaches to co-morbidity management for Western consumers. Chronic care needs to be proactive, consumer-oriented and multidisciplinary, which can be accessed by the people who need it most. Research is needed to identify how to facilitate seamless, coordinated and cost-effective care that improves outcomes for consumers with co-morbidities in their everyday lives within a supportive health-care system.

References

Aakvik, A., Holmas, T. (2006) Access to primary health care and health outcomes: the relationships between GP characteristics and mortality rates. *Journal of Health Economics* **25**(6): 1139–1153.

Aiken, L., Clarke, S., Sloane, D. (2002) Hospital staffing, organization, and quality of care: cross-national findings. *International Journal for Quality in Health Care* **14**(1): 5–13.

Alexander, G., Casalino, L., Meltzer, D. (2003) Patient-physician communication about out-of-pocket costs. *Journal of the American Medical Association* **290**(7): 953–958.

Alkema, G., Shannon, G., Wilber, K. (2003) Using interagency collaboration to serve older adults with chronic care needs: the care advocate program. *Family and Community Health* **26**(3): 221–229.

Anderson, M., Clarke, M., Helms, L., Foreman, M. (2005) Hospital readmission from home health care before and after prospective payment. *Journal of Nursing Scholarship* **37**(1): 73–79.

Armitage, S., Kavanagh, K. (1998) Consumer-oriented outcomes in discharge planning: a pilot study. *Journal of Clinical Nursing* **7**: 67–74.

Australian Institute of Health & Welfare. (2004) *Australian Hospital Statistics 2002–2003*. Canberra.

Badley, E., Glazier, R. (2004) *Arthritis and Related Conditions in Ontario: ICES Research Atlas*, 2nd edition. Institute for Clinical Evaluative Sciences: Toronto.

Badley, E., Veinot, P., Tyas, J. et al. (2007) *2006 Survey of Orthopaedic Surgeons in Ontario*, Working Paper (07–3). Arthritis Community Research & Evaluation Unit (ACREU): Toronto.

Bayliss, E., Bosworth, H., Noel, P., Wolff, J., Damush, T., McIver, L. (2007) Supporting self-management for patients with complex medical needs: recommendations of a working group. *Chronic Illness* 6(3): 167–175.

Blakeman, T., MacDonald, W., Bower, P., Gately, C., Chew-Graham, C. (2006) A qualitative study of GPs' attitudes to self-management of chronic disease. *British Journal of General Practice* 56(527): 407–414.

Bodenheimer, T., Lorig, K., Holman, H., Grumbach, K. (2002) Innovations in primary care. Patient self-management of chronic disease in primary care. *Journal of the American Medical Association* 288(19): 2469–2475.

Bouchard, M.-H., Dragomir, A., Blais, L., Berard, A., Pilon, D., Perreault, S. (2007) Impact of adherence to statins on coronary artery disease in primary prevention. *British Journal of Clinical Pharmacology* 63(6): 698–708.

Brailer, D., Kroch, E., Pauly, M., Huang, J. (1996) Comorbidity-adjusted complication risk: a new outcome quality measure. *Medical Care* 34(5): 490–505.

Brand, C., Jones, C., Lowe, A. et al. (2004) A transitional care service for elderly chronic disease patients at risk of readmission. *Australian Health Review* 28(30): 275–284.

Burton, C. (2000) Re-thinking stroke rehabilitation: the Corbin and Strauss chronic illness trajectory framework. *Journal of Advanced Nursing* 32(3): 595–602.

Cabana, M., Jee, S. (2004) Does continuity of care improve patient outcomes? *Journal of Family Practice* 53(12): 974–980.

Campbell, S., Hann, M., Hacker, J. et al. (2001) Identifying predictors of high quality care in English general practice: observational study. *British Medical Journal* 323(7316): 784–787.

Chan, L., Koepsell, T., Deyo, R. et al. (1997) The effect of Medicare's payment system for rehabilitation hospitals on length of stay, charges, and total payments. *New England Journal of Medicine* 337(14): 978–985.

Chodosh, J., Morton, S., Mojica, W. et al. (2005) Meta-analysis: chronic disease self-management programs for older adults. *Annals of Internal Medicine* 143(6): 427–438.

Cleary, P., Greenfield, S., Mulley, A. et al. (1991) Variations in length of stay and outcomes for six medical and surgical conditions in Massachusetts and California. *Journal of the American Medical Association* 266(1): 73–79.

Cohen-Kohler, J. (2007) The morally uncomfortable global drug gap. *Clinical Pharmacology and Therapeutics* 82(5): 610–614.

Colman, P., Thomas, D., Zimmet, P., Welborn, T., Garcia-Webb, P., Moore, M. (1999) New classification and criteria for diagnosis of diabetes mellitus: position statement. *Medical Journal of Australia* 170(8): 375–378.

Cooke, C., Fatodu, H. (2006) Physician conformity and patient adherence to ACE inhibitors and ARBs in patients with diabetes, with and without renal disease and hypertension, in a medicaid managed care organization. *The Journal of Managed Care Pharmacy* 12(8): 649–655.

Cooper, B., Yarmo Roberts, D. (2006) National case management standards in Australia – purpose, process and potential impact. *Australian Health Review* 30(1): 12–16.

Corbin, J.M., Strauss, A. (1991) A nursing model for chronic illness management based upon the trajectory framework. *Scholarly Inquiry for Nursing Practice* 5(3): 155–174.

de Crespigny, C., Emden, C., Drage, B., Hobby, C., Smith, S. (2002) Missed opportunities in the field: caring for clients with co-morbidity problems. *Collegian* **9**(3): 29–34.

Department of Human Services (DHS). (2007) *Mental Health & Drugs Matter Newsletter.* Melbourne, June 2007.

Diwan, S. (1999) Allocation of case management resources in long-term care: predicting high use of case management time. *Gerontologist* **39**(5): 580–590.

Doran, C., Chiarelli, P., Cockburn, J. (2001) Economic costs of urinary incontinence in community-dwelling Australian women. *Medical Journal of Australia* **174**(9): 456–458.

Duke, C. (2005) The frail elderly community-based case management project. *Geriatric Nursing* **26**(2): 122–127.

Dunbar-Jacob, J. (2007) Models for changing patient behaviour. *American Journal of Nursing* **107**(6): 20–25.

Dunlop, D., Semanik, P., Song, J., Manheim, L.M., Shih, V., Chang, R. (2005) Risk factors for functional decline in older adults with arthritis. *Arthritis and Rheumatism* **52**(4): 1274–1282.

Dunstan, D., Zimmett, P., Welborn, T. *et al.* (2002) The rising prevalence of diabetes and impaired glucose tolerance: the Australian diabetes, obesity and lifestyle study. *Diabetes Care* **25**(5): 829–834.

Feinstein, A. (1970) The pre-therapeutic classification of co-morbidity in chronic disease. *Journal of Chronic Diseases* **23**: 455–468.

Figar, S., Hornstein, L., Rada, M. *et al.* (2006) Effect of education on blood pressure control in elderly persons: a randomized controlled trial. *American Journal of Hypertension* **19**(7): 737–743.

Fortin, P., Penrod, J., Clarke, A. *et al.* (2002) Timing of total joint replacement affects clinical outcomes among patients with osteoarthritis of the hip or knee. *Arthritis and Rheumatism* **46**(12): 3327–3330.

Foster, N., Pincus, T., Underwood, M., Vogel, S., Breen, A., Harding, G. (2003) Understanding the process of care for musculoskeletal problems – why a biomedical approach is inadequate. *Rheumatology* **42**(3): 401–404.

Gagnon, A., Schein, C., McVey, L., Bergman, H. (1999) Randomized controlled trial of nurse case management of frail older people. *Journal of the American Geriatrics Society* **47**(9): 1118–1124.

Galbraith, A., Bullock, S., Manias, E., Hunt, B., Richards, A. (2007) *Fundamentals of Pharmacology*, 2nd edition. Pearson Education Limited: Essex.

Gallant, M. (2003) The influence of social support on chronic illness self-management: a review and directions for research. *Health Education and Behavior* **30**(2): 170–195, 248.

Garratt, A., Schmidt, L., Mackintosh, A., Fitzpatrick, R. (2002) Quality of life measurement: bibliographic study of patient assessed health outcome measures. *British Medical Journal* **324**(7351): 1417–1421.

Gask, L. (2005a) Role of specialists in common chronic diseases. *British Medical Journal* **330**(7492): 651–653.

Gask, L. (2005b) Is depression a chronic illness? For the motion. *Chronic Illness* **1**: 101–106.

Gately, C., Rogers, A., Sanders, C. (2007) Re-thinking the relationship between long-term condition self-management education and the utilisation of health services. *Social Sciences and Medicine*. Online 21 May 2007. DOI: 10.1016/j.socscimed. 2007.04.018.

Gignac, M., Cott, C. (1998) A conceptual model of independence and dependence for adults with chronic physical illness and disability. *Social Science and Medicine* **47**(6): 739–753.

Glanz, K., Rimer, B., Lewis, F. (2002) *Health Behavior and Health Education: Theory, Research and Practice*. John Wiley & Sons: San Francisco, CA.

Grant, R., Devita, N., Singer, D., Meigs, J. (2003) Polypharmacy and medication adherence in patients with Type 2 diabetes. *Diabetes Care* **26**(5): 1408–1412.

Gregg, E., Cheng, Y., Cadwell, B. *et al.* (2005) Secular trends in cardiovascular disease risk factors according to body mass index in US adults. *Journal of the American Medical Association* **293**(15): 1868–1874.

de Groot, V., Beckerman, H., Lankhorst, G., Bouter, L. (2003) How to measure comorbidity: a critical review of available methods. *Journal of Clinical Epidemiology* **56**: 221–229.

Gross, J., de Azevedo, M., Silveiro, S., Canani, L., Caramori, M., Zelmanovitz, T. (2005) Diabetic nephropathy: diagnosis, prevention, and treatment. *Diabetes Care* **28**(1): 164–176.

Hadjistavropoulos, H., Berlein, C., Sagan, M., Quine, A. (2003) Linking guidelines for case management to risk of institutionalization. *Case Management* **4**(4): 202–208.

Haggerty, J., Reid, R., Freeman, G., Starfield, B., Adair, C., McKendry, R. (2003) Continuity of care: a multidisciplinary review. *British Medical Journal* **327**(7425): 1219–1221.

Harris, M., Zwar, N. (2007) Care of patients with chronic disease: the challenge for general practice. *Medical Journal of Australia* **187**(2): 104–107.

Hawthorne, G., Osbourne, R. (2005) Population norms and meaningful differences for the assessment of quality of life (AQOL) measure. *Australian and New Zealand Journal of Public Health* **29**(2): 136–142.

Haynes, R., Yao, X., Degani, A., Kripalani, S., Garg, A., McDonald, H. (2005) Interventions for enhancing medication adherence. *Cochrane Database of Systematic Reviews* Issue 4: Art. No.: CD000011. DOI: 10.1002/14651858.

Hedges, G., Grimmer, K., Moss, J., Falco, J. (1999) Performance indicators for discharge planning: a focused review of the literature. *Australian Journal of Advanced Nursing* **16**(4): 20–28.

Hovenga, E. (1998) Organisational performance evaluation. In: Clinton, M., Scheiwe, D. (eds) *Management in the Australian Health Care Industry*, 2nd edition. Longman: South Melbourne, Australia, pp. 111–139.

Hu, T., Wagner, T., Bentkover, J., Leblanc, K., Zhou, S., Hunt, T. (2004) Costs of urinary incontinence and overactive bladder in the United States: a comparative study. *Urology* **63**(3): 461–465.

Jain, N.B., Guller, U., Pietrobon, R., Bond, T., Higgins, L. (2005) Comorbidities increase complication rates in patients having arthroplasty. *Clinical Orthopaedics and Related Research* **435**: 232–238.

Joachim, G., Acorn, S. (2000) Stigma of visible and invisible conditions. *Journal of Advanced Nursing* **32**(1): 243–248.

Johnson, M., Griffiths, R., Piper, M., Langdon, R. (2005) Risk factors for an untoward medication event among elders in community-based nursing caseloads in Australia. *Public Health Nursing* **22**(1): 36–44.

Kalsekar, I., Madhavan, S., Amonkar, M. *et al.* (2006) Depression in patients with type 2 diabetes: impact on adherence to oral hypoglycemic agents. *The Annals of Pharmacotherapy* **40**(4): 605–611.

Keener, J., Callaghan, J., Goetz, D., Pederson, D., Sullivan, P., Johnston, R. (2003) Twenty-five year results after Charnley total hip arthroplasty in patients less than fifty years old: a concise follow-up of a previous report. *Journal of Bone and Joint Surgery* **85A**(6): 1066–1072.

Kempen, G., Ormel, J., Brilman, E., Relyveld, J. (1997) Adaptive responses among Dutch elderly: the impact of eight chronic medical conditions on health-related quality of life. *American Journal of Public Health* **87**(1): 38–44.

Kennedy, A., Lee, V., Gardner, C. (2007) The effectiveness and cost effectiveness of a national lay-led self care support programme for patients with long-term conditions: a pragmatic randomised controlled trial. *Journal of Epidemiology and Community Health* **61**(3): 254–261.

Kinney, E., Kennedy, J., Cook, C., Freedman, J., Lane, K., Hui, S. (2003) A randomized trial of two quality improvement strategies implemented in a statewide public community-based, long-term care program. *Medical Care* **41**(9): 1048–1057.

Kozma, C. (1998) Disease management: the role of comorbidities in disease state management. *Managed Care Interface* **11**(7): 65–66.

Kralik, D. (2002) The quest for ordinariness: transition experienced by midlife women living with chronic illness. *Journal of Advanced Nursing* **39**(2): 146–154.

Kralik, D., Seymour, L., Eastwood, S., Koch, T. (2007) Managing the self: living with an indwelling urinary catheter. *Journal of Nursing and Healthcare of Chronic Illness* **16**(7b): 177–185.

Kripalani, S., Yao, X., Haynes, R. (2007) Interventions to enhance medication adherence in chronic medical conditions: a systematic review. *Archives of Internal Medicine* **167**(6): 540–550.

Krumholz, H., Amatruda, J., Smith, G. *et al.* (2002) Randomized trial of an education and support intervention to prevent readmission of patients with heart failure. *Journal of the American College of Cardiology* **39**(1): 83–89.

Krumholz, H., Currie, P., Riegel, B. *et al.* (2006) A taxonomy for disease management: a scientific statement from the American Heart Association Disease Management Taxonomy Writing Group. *Circulation* **114**(13): 1432–1445.

Lapsley, H., March, L., Tribe, K., Cross, M., Brooks, P. (2001) Living with osteoarthritis: patient expenditures, health status, and social impact. *Arthritis Care and Research* **45**(3): 301–306.

Laukkanen, P., Sakari-Rantala, R., Kauppinen, M., Heikkinen, E. (1997) Morbidity and disability in 75- and 80-year old men and women: a five year follow-up. *Scandinavian Journal of Social Medicine* **53** (Suppl): 79–106.

Lawrence, D. (2002) *Can the NHS Learn from the USA? The Kaiser Permanente Experience of Integrated Care.* The 9th Annual Office of Health Economics Lecture Delivered by David Lawrence MD, Chairman and Chief Executive Officer of Kaiser Permanente: London.

Lee, D., Donovan, L., Austin, P. *et al.* (2005) Comparison of coding heart failure and comorbidities in administrative and clinical data for use in outcomes research. *Medical Care* **43**(2): 182–188.

Leucht, S., Burkard, T., Henderson, J., Maj, M., Sartorius, N. (2007) Physical illness and schizophrenia: a review of the literature. *Acta Psychiatrica Scandinavica* **116**: 317–333.

Levin, A., Stevens, L., McCullough, P. (2002) Cardiovascular disease and the kidney: tracking a killer in chronic kidney disease. *Postgraduate Medicine* **111**(4) Online. Viewed 12 November 2006, http://www.postgradmed.com/issues.

Lindenmeyer, A., Van Royen, P., Wens, J., Hearnshaw, H., Vermeire, E., Biot, Y. (2006) Interventions to improve adherence to medication in people with type 2 diabetes mellitus: a review of the literature on the role of pharmacists. *Journal of Clinical Pharmacy and Therapeutics* **31**(5): 409–419.

Linn, B.S., Linn, M.W., Gurel, L. (1968) Cumulative illness rating scale. *Journal of the American Geriatrics Society* **16**(5): 662–666.

Long, L., Mann, R. (1998) Casemix: challenges for nursing care. *Medical Journal of Australia* **169** (Suppl.): S44–S45.

Lorig, K., Ritter, P., Laurent, D., Fries, J. (2004) Long-term randomized controlled trials of tailored-print and small-group arthritis self-management interventions. *Medical Care* **42**(4): 346–354.

Lorig, K., Ritter, P., Stewart, A. *et al.* (2001) Chronic disease self-management program: 2 year health status and health care utilization outcomes. *Medical Care* **39**(1): 1217–1223.

Lorig, K.R., Sobel, D.S., Stewart, A.L. *et al.* (1999) Evidence suggesting that a chronic disease self-management program can improve health status while reducing hospitalization: a randomised trial. *Medical Care* **37**(1): 5–14.

Lubkin, I., Larsen, P. (eds) (2002) *Chronic Illness: Impact and Interventions*, 5th edition. Jones & Bartlett: Boston, MA.

MacLennan, W. (1998) Caring for carers. *Age and Ageing* **27**(5): 651–652.

McCormick, W., Kukull, W., van Belle, G., Bowen, J., Teri, L., Larson, E. (1994) Symptom patterns and comorbidity in the early stages of Alzheimer's disease. *Journal of the American Geriatrics Society* **42**(5): 517–521.

McGann, P. (2000) Comorbidity in heart failure in the elderly. *Clinics in Geriatric Medicine* **16**(3): 631–648.

McMurray, A., Grant, S., Griffiths, S., Letford, A. (2002) Health-related quality of life and health service use following total hip replacement surgery. *Journal of Advanced Nursing* **40**(6): 663–672.

Miller, J. (1992) *Coping with Chronic Illness: Overcoming Powerlessness*, 2nd edition. F.A. Davis Company: Philadelphia, PA.

Miller, M., Paradis, C., Houck, P. *et al.* (1992) Rating chronic medical illness burden in geropsychiatric practice and research: application of the cumulative illness rating scale. *Psychiatry Research* **41**: 237–248.

Morse, J. (1997) Responding to threats to integrity of self. *Advances in Nursing Science* **19**(4): 21–36.

Murray, E., Burns, J., See Tai, S., Lai, R., Nazareth, I. (2005) Interactive health communication applications for people with chronic disease. *Cochrane Database of Systematic Reviews* Reviews Issue 4: Art. No.: CD004274. DOI: 10.1002/14651858.

Murray-Johnson, L., Witte, K., Boulay, M., Figueroa, M.E., Storey, D., Tweedie, I. (2000) Using health education theories to explain behavior change: a cross-country analysis. *International Quarterly of Community Health Education* **20**(4): 323–345.

Nader, C. (2007) The despair of living with an illness that has no home. *The Age Newspaper* 2.

Naicker, S. (2003) End-stage renal disease in sub-Saharan and South Africa. *Kidney International* 63: 119–122.

Nardi, R., Scanelli, G., Corrao, S., Iori, I., Mathieu, G., Amatrian, R. (2007) Co-morbidity does not reflect complexity in internal medicine patients. *European Journal of Internal Medicine* 18(5): 359–368.

Nay, R., Garratt, S., Koch, S. (1999) Challenges for Australian nursing in the international year of older persons. *Geriatric Nursing* 20(1): 14–17.

Newbould, J., Taylor, D., Bury, M. (2006) Lay-led self-management in chronic disease: a review of the literature. *Chronic Illness* 2(4): 249–261.

Papenhausen, J., Escandon-Dominguez, S., Michaels, C. (1998) Nurse case management. In: Lubkin, I.M., Larsen, P.D. (eds) *Chronic Illness: Impact and Interventions*, 4th edition. Jones & Bartlett: Boston, MA, pp. 453–474.

Parker, J. (1999) Patient or customer? Caring practices in nursing and the global supermarket of care. *Collegian* 6(1): 16–23.

Parris, E., Lawrence, D., Mohn, L., Long, L. (2005) Adherence to statin therapy and LDL cholesterol goal attainment by patients with diabetes and dyslipidemia. *Diabetes Care* 28(3): 595–599.

Parry-Jones, B., Soulsby, J. (2001) Needs-led assessment: the challenges and the reality. *Health and Social Care in the Community* 9(6): 414–428.

Paterson, B. (2001) The shifting perspectives model of chronic illness. *Journal of Nursing Scholarship* 33(1): 21–26.

Paterson, B., Russell, C., Thorne, S. (2001) Critical analysis of everyday self-care decision making in chronic illness. *Journal of Advanced Nursing* 35(3): 335–341.

Paterson, B., Thorne, S., Russell, C. (2002) Disease-specific influences on meaning and significance in self-care decision-making in chronic illness. *Canadian Journal of Nursing Research* 34(3): 61–74.

Pfeiffer, D. (2000) The devils are in the details: the ICIDH2 and the disability movement. *Disability and Society* 15(7): 1079–1082.

Picavet, H.S., Hoeymans, N. (2004) Health-related quality of life in multiple musculoskeletal diseases: SF-36 and EQ-5D in the DMC3 study. *Annals of the Rheumatic Diseases* 63(6): 723–729.

Poulton, B. (1999) User involvement in identifying health needs and shaping and evaluating services: is it being realised? *Journal of Advanced Nursing* 30(6): 1289–1296.

Pound, P., Yardley, L., Campbell, R. *et al.* (2005) Resisting medicines: a synthesis of qualitative studies of medicine taking. *Social Science and Medicine* 61(1): 133–155.

Powell, A., Teichtahl, A., Wluka, A., Cicuttini, F. (2005) Obesity: a preventable risk factor for large joint osteoarthritis which may act through biomechanical factors. *British Journal of Sports Medicine* 39(1): 4–5.

Proctor, E., Morrow-Howell, N., Kaplan, S. (1996) Implementation of discharge plans for chronically ill elders discharged home. *Health and Social Work* 21(1): 30–40.

Raddish, M., Horn, S.D., Sharkey, P.D. (1999) Continuity of care: is it cost effective? *American Journal of Managed Care* 5(6): 727–734.

Redelmeier, D., Tan, S., Booth, G. (1998) The treatment of unrelated disorders in patients with chronic medical diseases. *New England Journal of Medicine* 338(21): 1516–1520.

Rijken, M., van Kerkhof, M., Dekker, J., Schellevis, F. (2005) Comorbidity of chronic diseases: effects of disease pairs on physical and mental functioning. *Quality of Life Research* **14**(1): 45–55.

Rolland, J. (1987) Chronic illness and the life-cycle - a conceptual framework. *Family Process* **26**(2): 203–221.

Roter, D., Hall, J., Merisca, R., Nordstrom, B., Cretin, D., Svarstad, B. (1998) Effectiveness of interventions to improve patient compliance: a meta-analysis. *Medical Care* **36**(8): 1138–1161.

Rothman, A., Wagner, E. (2003) Chronic illness management: what is the role of primary care? *Annals of Internal Medicine* **138**(3): 256–261.

Rudy, T., Weiner, D., Lieber, S., Slaboada, J., Boston, J. (2007) The impact of chronic low back pain on older adults: a comparative study of patients and controls. *Pain* **131**: 293–301.

Rutledge, D., Donaldson, N., Pravikoff, D. (2001) End-of-life care series, Part II: end-of-life care for hospitalized adults in America-learnings from the SUPPORT and HELP studies. *Online Journal of Clinical Innovations* **4**: 1–57.

Rycroft-Malone, J., Latter, S., Yerill, P. (2001) Consumerism in health care: the case of medication education. *Journal of Nursing Management* **9**: 221–230.

Saltman, D. (2005) Co-morbidity issues are still overlooked. *Medical Observer* (10th June), 18.

Schifalacqua, M., Hook, M., O'Hearn, P., Schmidt, M. (2000) Coordinating the care of the chronically ill in a world of managed care. *Nursing Administration Quarterly* **24**(3): 12–20.

Schirm, V. (2002) Quality of life. In: Lubkin, I.M., Larsen, P.D. (eds) *Chronic Illness: Impact and Interventions*, 5th edition. Jones & Bartlett: Boston, MA, pp. 181–201.

Schroeder, K., Fahey, T., Hay, A., Montgomery, A., Peters, T., Ebrahim, S. (2006) Relationship between medication adherence and blood pressure in primary care: prospective study. *Journal of Human Hypertension* **20**(8): 625–627.

Sequist, T., Gandhi, T., Karson, A. *et al.* (2005) A randomized trial of electronic clinical reminders to improve quality of care for diabetes and coronary artery disease. *Journal of the American Medical Informatics Association* **12**(4): 431–437.

Smith, P., Araya-Guerra, R., Bublitz, C. *et al.* (2005) Missing clinical information during primary care visits. *Journal of the American Medical Association* **293**(5): 565–571.

Smith, S., O'Dowd, T. (2007) Chronic diseases: what happens when they come in multiples? *British Journal of General Practice* **57**(537): 268–270.

Sparbel, K., Anderson, M. (2000) Integrated literature review of continuity of care: Part 1, conceptual issues. *Journal of Nursing Scholarship* **32**(1): 17–24.

Sprangers, M., de Regt, E., Andries, F. *et al.* (2000) Which chronic conditions are associated with better or poorer quality of life? *Journal of Clinical Epidemiology* **53**(9): 895–907.

Steinbrook, R. (1998) Patients with multiple chronic conditions – how many medications are enough? [Editorial]. *New England Journal of Medicine* **338**(21): 1541–1542.

Stevenson, F., Cox, K., Britten, N., Dundar, Y. (2004) A systematic review of the research on communication between patients and health care professionals about medicines: the consequences for concordance. *Health Expectations* **7**(3): 235–245.

Stone, R. (2004) The direct care worker: the third rail of home care policy. *Annual Review of Public Health* **25**: 521–537.

Temmink, D., Francke, A., Hutten, J., van der Zee, J., Abu-Saad, H. (2000) Innovations in the nursing care of the chronically ill: a literature review from an international perspective. *Journal of Advanced Nursing* **31**(6): 1449–1458.

Thomas, M., Atkins, R. (2006) Blood pressure lowering for the prevention and treatment of diabetic kidney disease. *Drugs* **66**(17): 2213–2234.

Townsend, A., Wyke, S., Hunt, K. (2006) Self-managing and managing self: practical and moral dilemmas in accounts of living with chronic illness. *Chronic Illness* **2**: 185–194.

Vale, M., Jelinek, M., Best, J. *et al.* (2003) Coaching patients on achieving cardiovascular health (COACH): a multicenter randomized trial in patients with coronary heart disease. *Archives of Internal Medicine* **163**(22): 2775–2783.

Vas, J., Mendez, C., Perea-Milla, E. *et al.* (2004) Acupuncture as a complementary therapy to the pharmacological treatment of osteoarthritis of the knee: randomised controlled trial. *British Medical Journal* **329**(7476): 1216–1221.

Verbrugge, L., Lepkowski, J., Imanaka, Y. (1989) Comorbidity and its impact on disability. *Milbank Quarterly* **67**(3–4): 450–484.

Verbrugge, L., Patrick, D. (1995) Seven chronic conditions: their impact on US adults' activity levels and use of medical services. *American Journal of Public Health* **85**(2): 173–182.

Verbrugge, L., Reoma, J., Gruber-Baldini, A. (1994) Short-term dynamics of disability and well-being. *Journal of Health and Social Behavior* **35**: 97–117.

Vermeire, E., Wens, J., Van Royen, P., Biot, Y., Hearnshaw, H., Lindenmeyer, A. (2005) Interventions for improving adherence to treatment recommendations in people with type 2 diabetes mellitus. *Cochrane Database of Systematic Reviews* Issue 2: Art. No.: CD003638. DOI:10.1002/14651858.CD003638.pub2.

Wagner, E.H., Davis, C., Schaefer, J., Von Korff, M., Austin, B. (2002) A survey of leading chronic disease management programs: are they consistent with the literature? *Journal of Nursing Care Quality* **16**(2): 67–80.

Walker, A. (2005) *Multiple Chronic Conditions: Patient Characteristics and Impacts on Quality of Life and Health Expenditure.* Health Services and Policy Research Conference, Canberra.

Ward, R. (1990) Health care provider choice and satisfaction. In: Stahl, S.M. (ed.) *The Legacy of Longevity: Health and Heath Care in Later Life.* Sage Publication: Newbury Park, CA, pp. 273–290.

Ware, J.E., Bayliss, M.S., Rogers, W.H., Kosinski, M., Tarlov, A.R. (1996) Differences in 4-year health outcomes for elderly and poor, chronically ill patients treated in HMO and fee-for-service systems: results from the medical outcomes study. *Journal of the American Medical Association* **276**(13): 1039–1047.

Wellard, S. (1998) Constructions of chronic illness. *International Journal of Nursing Studies* **35**(1–2): 49–55.

Williams, A. (2004) Patients with comorbidities: perceptions of acute care services. *Journal of Advanced Nursing* **46**(1): 13–22.

Williams, A., Botti, M. (2002) Issues concerning the on-going care of patients with comorbidities in acute care and post-discharge in Australia: a literature review. *Journal of Advanced Nursing* **40**(2): 131–140.

Williams, A., Dunning, T., Manias, E. (2007) Continuity of care and general wellbeing of patients with comorbidities requiring joint replacement: an Australian study. *Journal of Advanced Nursing* **57**(3): 244–256.

World Health Organization. (2003) In: Sabaté, E. (ed.) *Adherence to Long-term Therapies: Evidence for Action*. World Health Organization: Geneva, pp. 1–209.

Wright, S., Walsh, H., Ingley, K. *et al.* (2003) Uptake of self-management strategies in a heart failure management programme. *European Journal of Heart Failure* **5**(3): 371–380.

Zochling, J., March, L., Lapsley, H., Cross, M., Tribe, K., Brooks, P. (2004) Use of complementary medicines for osteoarthritis – a prospective study. *Annals of the Rheumatic Diseases* **63**(5): 549–554.

5. Conceptualisation of Self-Management

Malcolm Battersby, Sharon Lawn and Rene Pols

Introduction

The number one health policy priority facing many national governments is the cost and morbidity associated with chronic diseases or 'chronic conditions' [The WHO definition of 'chronic condition' is broad and includes HIV/AIDS, tuberculosis, cardiovascular disease, diabetes and long-term mental illness (World Health Organization 2002)]. This has led to increasing focus on the role of the people with chronic conditions in the management of their own health. Consideration of what constitutes self-management begins with the recognition that people with chronic conditions live their lives in spite of their symptoms and disabilities. For most people, the condition is not their first priority or focus and everyday they make decisions that affect the management of their chronic conditions without advice from health professionals. Previous generations of health professionals have been trained to diagnose, investigate and provide treatment or management, that is 'heal the sick' who are acutely ill. The focus on the prevention and management of chronic conditions has led to a re-examination of the role of the health professional, the practice and the health system in assisting the person to manage his/her condition(s).

All people learn from an early stage of life to be involved in their own self-care. Most people learn the essential principles of health and hygiene but few understand the many complexities associated with reducing or minimising personal health risks. Many people have widely divergent, culturally influenced beliefs and expectations about health, illness and what to do to optimise personal health outcomes. So also, when people develop risk factors for disease and are in the early stages of ill health, they often have unhelpful beliefs, attitudes and behaviours in respect of diet, health behaviours and ways in which they access the health system.

The compliance literature shows that few people consistently follow the directions of health practitioners and that many use unproven approaches to health issues (Vermeire *et al.* 2001). This is especially concerning in people from culturally diverse backgrounds where communication among the patient, carer and health professionals may be more challenging because of communication difficulties from both the service recipient and worker perspective, especially where cultural perspectives are misunderstood and where interpreters are not used effectively.

There is clear evidence that some people are excessively focused on their self-care and spend unnecessary time and resources to deal with problems or conditions that have no simple evidence-based answers. Yet, such people can be heavy users of the health-care system. There are also many people who are less focused on their self-care. This is evidenced by the failure of many people in developed countries to address their risk factors for health, in particular attending to their levels of exercise and weight. There are many systems of beliefs and ideas about what constitutes 'health', 'illnesses' and 'risk factors for health'. There are complementary medicines and natural therapies that comprise a substantial industry and impact on self-care. Paterson and Hopwood (see Chapter 6) discuss this phenomenon in the context of the rise of 'healthism', especially within Western neo-liberal economies. Individual behaviour, attitudes and emotions are viewed as 'factors that need attention for the realisation of health, and solutions to preventing or managing illness are seen to lie in the realm of individual choice'. Within this view, personal responsibility is paramount. Behaviours, attitudes and emotions are medicalised and people become morally accountable for their health choices and are at risk of being blamed and stigmatised for their choices.

Self-care is everything that people do to maintain life and satisfy their needs including activities of daily living such as washing, dressing, being educated and communicating with others. These activities may or may not have an impact on health, the development of risk factors for chronic conditions or on established chronic conditions. It is therefore pragmatic to use the term self-management to separately describe those activities that a person does that directly impact on risk factors or established chronic conditions. Self-management is a component of self-care that is informed by evidence-based health information.

The term *chronic condition self-management* ('self-management') has emerged as a concept to describe the tasks, roles and responsibilities of individuals as they cope with their chronic conditions from diagnosis to their long-term management. This chapter will provide international, historical and policy contexts to self-management – describing associated concepts that overlap with or inform an understanding of self-management from both the person's and the health professional's perspective. It will also describe the development of self-management concepts and practical applications of these, including nationally accepted definitions of self-management in Australia.

Background to the use of the term self-management

The individual's perspective

There is little explicit recognition that being diagnosed with a chronic illness is a critical life event for the individual. Such a crisis has well-defined characteristics (Caplan 1964; Gunderson & Rahe 1974). Put simply, it is a time of emotional disequilibrium and one that needs resolution through the learning of new skills to cope with the challenge that is presented. Once the challenge is confronted, dealt with and overcome, the person achieves a sense of mastery, and self-efficacy grows (Bandura 1977). This is the first step in developing an effective self-management approach to any clinical condition.

The person's experience of chronic illness is subjective, interpersonal and social. Self-management tasks involve an understanding of and distinguishing between the illness experiences, levels of distress, perceived loss of well-being, illness behaviour and the impaired functioning observed by others. Optimal self-management has the potential to also reduce the effects of the conditions or diseases on the person, such as social stigma and exclusion, and increase levels of participation in the family and community. Self-management tasks promote full personal and social well-being. Likewise, the carer's perspective is unique. It involves the impact that caring for someone with chronic illness has on the carer's role, interpersonal relationships with the person and others as well as their own careers and lives (Australian Bureau of Statistics 2003).

Individuals with a chronic condition tend to associate chronic illness with preventable diseases (Walker *et al.* 2003, p. 211). This is particularly so in Western cultures, though not in all cultures. For example, one of the problems among Aboriginal people in Canada is that they view diabetes as inevitable and unpreventable (Benyshek 2005). The disease prevention perspective has tended to view the treatment of chronic conditions as part of a disease model with the professional as the 'expert'. Within this traditional medical model, health is defined as the absence of disease. Solutions are usually sought within a medical context with the 'expert' health professional given primary responsibility for solutions. Such solutions are often described in a medical care plan. However, holistic patient-centred care can only be said to be achieved if there is a comprehensive integrated care plan that has been developed collaboratively between the patient, carer and/or family, doctor and other involved health workers – one that recognises the social context in which people live within their community. Different models will have direct impacts on service delivery to people with chronic illness, how self-management, control and responsibility for this is perceived and whether it serves to marginalise and stigmatise or empower the person. Walker and colleagues call for a definition that incorporates a greater understanding of social and cultural factors in which chronic conditions are experienced (Walker *et al.* 2003, p. 213). Within this definition, the distinction between chronic condition and chronic disease is an important one. A person may have a chronic condition, such as blindness or paraplegia, which presents as a disability that has the potential to remain static throughout the person's life. In contrast to this, chronic disease has the potential to be progressive because of an active disease process.

A public health perspective

Between the 1950s and 1970s, the development of health education and health promotion approaches emerged in response to a dissatisfaction with the disease model. Behavioural and environmental approaches emerged with a series of initiatives that would exert a major influence on how health and illness were perceived. The Alma Ata Declaration of 1977 was committed to 'health for all' via community participation and inter-sectoral collaboration. The Ottawa Charter of Health Promotion (World Health Organization 1986), incorporating a sociological and ecological analysis of health and disease increasingly recognised the role played by social determinants such as poverty and unemployment on health and attempted to address the problem of 'victim-blaming' or 'parent blaming' that had been a feature of earlier individualistic approaches. Understanding the role of social determinants of health across the lifespan is a view that recognises that ways of coping, behaving and self-efficacy notions are intertwined with experiences and exposures throughout the lifecycle, not just once the person becomes unwell. The role of socialisation, culture and economic circumstances helps to explain how the experience of chronic illness and the resources available for its self-management may vary between individuals and groups of individuals.

A mental health perspective

In the mental health sector self-management is embedded in the notion of 'recovery' and there is a strong psychosocial focus that understands that the person's circumstances are due to a complex range of elements within the person and the environment (Brooks 2002; Pepper 2002; Davidson 2004). As part of this, addressing stigma and enhancing empowerment are significant objectives. What a person needs in order to exist (core needs) versus what a person needs in order to flourish (respect and dignity regardless of level of disability) are discussed at length by Ignatieff (1994). Such notions lie at the core of self-management goals that people hold for themselves. They are about optimising wellness or well-being, not necessarily achieving complete cure. They involve, but are not limited to, the protection and promotion of health and well-being by

- being able to make and participate in informed decisions;
- building and sustaining partnerships with others;
- being able to manage the impacts of illness; and
- monitoring and managing symptoms and signs of illness/chronic conditions (Whitby 2003).

Historical developments in self-management

Wilcocks (2001), in her history of occupational therapy, argues that self-management with guidance from 'expert' health professionals goes back to medieval times in the form of the 'Regimen Sanitatis' where recommendations for preventive self-management for general and personal use were described discursively as well as in tabular forms (p. 119). In more recent times, the self-help movement had its origins after the First World War in the rehabilitation of amputee and blinded veterans who were encouraged to live effectively in spite of their disability. In a more therapeutic way the management of tuberculosis also had behavioural self-management as a significant component of care. The first self-help organisation was in fact Alcoholics Anonymous, which has provided the foundation for modern self-management approaches to the management of chronic conditions since the 1930s (Alcoholics Anonymous 2007).

The addiction field has offered clear examples of the development of self-management and self-management support with the rise of self-help groups such as Alcoholic Anonymous and its related groups for other drugs of addiction and addictive behaviours such as gambling. In addition, it recognised the importance of the roles of carers involved with the patient by providing education and support for them also (e.g. Alanon and Naranon). The self-help model stresses that each person with a chronic condition can also be a helper to others. It emphasises the helper's role and how this promotes greater independence and less dependence, and how it helps the person to put their own problems in perspective, giving the helper a sense of social usefulness by adopting a helping role (Riessman & Carroll 1995). Mutual aid models such as this are not new. Like the field of occupational therapy, they abound in the history and development of the social work profession (Shulman 1992). There is now a plethora of self-help organisations for hundreds of issues and conditions, with a proliferation of self-help media through self-help books and websites.

More recently, disease-specific approaches to self-management have been led by diabetes, arthritis, asthma and cardiac academics, clinicians and self-help organisations. Diabetes has been an exemplar in defining the roles of the individual in the self-management of their condition through the development of an education curriculum (American Diabetes Association). This education has been delivered through the role of the diabetes educator (Funnell & Anderson 2004). Similarly, the role of asthma educators, arthritis self-management programmes and cardiac rehabilitation practitioners has been established in most developed countries. These disease-specific education programmes have usually been provided in both group and face-to-face format.

After initial enthusiasm for these programmes, research showed that education that provided information alone was largely ineffective in improving patient outcomes (Gibson *et al.* 2004). Gaining education and knowledge is an important component of self-management though not effective on its own. Effective education and knowledge of one's condition is dependent on several social factors including the following:

- Literacy level
- Access to resources – physical, social, financial
- Distance/isolation from supports and adequate resources
- Quality and availability of technology and media
- Culture and tradition
- Adherence

More recent developments therefore have defined the skills required for effective self-management, both, at a disease-specific level and those that are common (generic) to many chronic conditions (Lorig & Holman 2003a). Many of these skills are derived from cognitive and behavioural approaches to psychological problems (Bandura *et al.* 1977). Strategies that include a behaviour/skill component within a structured programme have been found to be more successful than education alone for people with chronic conditions (Connors 2005).

A cognitive behavioural therapy (CBT) approach to self-management is fundamentally linked with a crisis intervention model that recognises that a crisis offers a unique opportunity for the person to make positive change (Golan 1974). It also involves an important personal, emotional, social and spiritual adjustment and progress towards self-management, beyond the limits of a bio-psychosocial understanding (Drew 1987; Miller 1990). Medical practitioners, nurses and allied health workers are critical partners for patients faced with the diagnosis of any chronic condition. At the point of diagnosis, patients, doctors and health workers must join together as partners to develop complementary roles in the total management of the condition.

The biomedical, bio-psychosocial and behavioural models of chronic illness have also been useful in understanding how self-management is to be defined. The biomedical model sees chronic illness as 'persistent, unexplained, of indeterminate diagnosis or relapsing' (Walker *et al.* 2003, p. 210). Bio-psychosocial models aim to understand the complex relationship between biological disease paths, internal psychological forces within the person and external forces within their social environment. Behavioural models tend to leave out socio-economic factors.

The Stanford model of chronic disease self-management, developed by Lorig and colleagues in the 1970s (Lorig 1993), has also been prominent. It is based on problems perceived by the patient. The goal is to build the person's confidence (self-efficacy) to perform the three tasks of disease, role and emotional management, similarly defined by the Center for the Advancement of Health and Center for Health Studies Group Health Cooperative of Puget Sound (1996), with the end goal of improved health status and appropriate utilisation of health care. It draws heavily from the work of Corbin and Strauss (1988) in their earlier work with people with chronic conditions. They outline three tasks of self-management that people need to achieve in order to maintain 'wellness', rather than 'illness', in their psychological foreground as discussed by Lorig and Holman (2003a,2003b):

1. 'medical management of the condition.
2. maintaining, changing and creating new meaningful behaviours in life roles.
3. [dealing] with the emotional sequelae of having a chronic condition, which alters ones' view of the future' (p. 1).

Lorig and Holman also stress that 'self-management is a lifetime task' (2003b, p. 1) that acknowledges the patients as ultimately responsible for the day-to-day management of their condition (Lorig & Holman 2003a). The Stanford Model outlines six skills for self-management:

- Problem-solving.
- Decision-making.
- Resource utilisation – not just telling people about resources, but teaching them how to use them (may have significant implications for special populations who have traditionally had access issues regarding available resources).

- The formation of a patient–provider partnership – the professional is teacher and partner, not provider of diagnosis and treatment alone.
- Action planning.
- Self-tailoring – applying self-management skills and knowledge to the person's individual context.

More recently, definitions of self-management have been informed by the Chronic Care Model (Wagner *et al.* 2001). This model, derived from evidence, describes the six core elements in a practice or system of care that provide optimal prevention and management of chronic conditions for a population. These elements are provided by the health-care organisation and include self-management support. The aim of the six elements is to improve health outcomes for the individual by supporting the individual to become 'activated'. Figure 5.1 articulates the Chronic Care Model.

Each domain within the Chronic Care Model is described below.

Self-Management   Effective self-management is very different from telling patients what to do. Patients have a central role in determining their care, one that fosters a sense of responsibility for their own health.

Decision Support   Treatment decisions need to be based on explicit, proven guidelines supported by at least one defining study. Health-care organisations creatively integrate explicit, proven guidelines into the day-to-day practice of the primary care providers in an accessible and easy-to-use manner.

Delivery System Design   The delivery of patient care requires not only determining what care is needed, but also clarifying roles and tasks to ensure that the patient gets the care; making sure that all the clinicians who take care of a patient

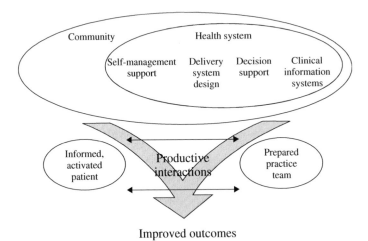

Figure 5.1   The Chronic Care Model. Source: Wagner, E.H. (1998) Chronic disease management: what will it take to improve care for chronic illness? *Effective Clinical Practice* **1**(1): 2–4. Reproduced with permission of the American College of Physicians.

have centralised, up-to-date information about the patient's status; and making follow-up a part of standard procedure.

Clinical Information System   A registry – an information system that can track individual patients as well as populations of patients – is a necessity when managing chronic illness or preventive care.

Organisation of Health Care   Health-care systems can create an environment in which organised efforts to improve the care of people with chronic illness take hold and flourish.

Community   To improve the health of the population health-care organisations reach out to form powerful alliances and partnerships with state programmes, local agencies, schools, faith organisations, businesses and clubs.

(The Chronic Care Model was developed by Ed Wagner, MD, MPH, Director of the MacColl Institute for Healthcare Innovation, Group Health Cooperative of Puget Sound and colleagues of the Improving Chronic Illness Care programme. This content from the Institute for Healthcare Improvement website (www.ihi.org) is reprinted with permission.)

Associated concepts or models that overlap with or inform self-management

When self-management is discussed a number of related themes can be identified from the literature, which help to understand how self-management should be defined so that it acknowledges the diversity of needs and populations with chronic conditions.

The person as expert

The notion of the person as expert recognises that the person is already self-managing to some extent, regardless of any input from others. The person as expert acknowledges that there are internal and external barriers to self-management that are amenable to change with self-management support, education, policy change and innovation. It is linked to resilience and locus of control notions as well as health beliefs and understandings from the person's perspective (Gunderson & Rahe 1974). This definition of 'expert' involves knowledge and understanding that is based on experience, not education (Wilson 2001). This view acknowledges the persons and their meanings, that the 'self' must be the central focus of self-management. The mistaken assumption of traditional health-care relationships is that the ideal expert patient is both compliant and self-reliant (Thorne *et al.* 2000; Wilson 2001). However, Horne and Weinman (1999) stress that 'people's own beliefs about medicines are known to be the most important determinant of whether medicines are taken ... [and that] doctors are not necessarily best placed to understand the realities of life for many of their patients' (Shaw & Baker 2004, p. 724).

Currently, the traditional methods of health-care delivery in developed and many developing countries foster the view that the health professional or doctor is the 'expert' and that the patient is a dependent recipient. As a response to this the National Health Service (NHS) in the United Kingdom has funded the provision of the Stanford chronic disease self-management course under the name 'Expert Patient Program'. Established in 2002, the NHS plans to provide this programme to 100,000 people with long-term conditions by 2012. The effectiveness of this programme has been the subject of much debate and has led to the seeking of alternative models. It has been variously challenged for its evidence base, for overstating the evidence for effectiveness, and for concerns regarding participation rates and perceived bias about the types of people who effectively engage in this model as those who are already well engaged with their own health self-management (Battersby 2006; Newbould *et al.* 2006). Its greatest criticism is that it is not reaching the most disadvantaged who have a disproportionate load on their health and are in greatest need of self-management skills. However, this is arguably not a problem with the programme as much as a problem with the health professionals' attitudes and selection bias as part of recruiting and promoting this approach to their patients. A growing number of studies clearly demonstrate that significantly disadvantaged groups do engage effectively in this and other self-management programmes (Lawn *et al.* 2007; Harvey *et al.* 2008). Caution is called for in the over-reliance on one approach to the exclusion of other ways of supporting people with self-management tasks (Rogers 2006).

An overlapping concept with the expert patient in the United Kingdom has been that of patient engagement. The Wanless report (Wanless 2002) argued that a viable health system needed to be 'fully engaged' with the public working alongside the health system to maximise their health. The NHS-commissioned research showed that patient's involvement in shared decision-making and self-management results in increased patient satisfaction, reduced anxiety, increased clinician satisfaction and improved individual patient health outcomes (Farrell 2004, p. 5). Further UK policy developments in the area of clinician education to support self-management have been informed by the Kings Fund review (Corben & Rosen 2005, p. 11), which recommended improving health profession-als' skills to support self-management, improving the provision of information about long-term conditions and the local services available and increasing the flexibility of service provision to fit in with patients' other commitments.

Empowerment

Effective self-management for people with chronic conditions includes empow-ering people to take responsibility for their evidence-based care. This includes providing them with optimal evidence-based interventions and knowledge and facilitating their effective engagement with self-management tasks (Wagner *et al.* 1996; Creer & Christian 1976). Hamman *et al.* (2003) argue that at least 50% of patients, including those with mental illness, are ready and willing to discuss and share decision-making with doctors; however, less than 10% of such decisions clearly include patients. Funnell *et al.* (1991) have developed an empowerment programme for diabetes care. Based on the training of health professionals, the *process of empowerment* is defined as 'the discovery and development of one's inher-ent capacity to be responsible for one's own life. People are empowered when they have sufficient knowledge, to make rational decisions, sufficient control and resources to implement their decisions and sufficient experience to evaluate the effectiveness of their decisions'. There is good evidence from randomised controlled trials that patient-centred interventions that actively involve patients in problem-solving and decision-making are especially beneficial for increasing participation, lowering decisional conflict and increasing knowledge (Anderson *et al.* 1995; Roter *et al.* 1998).

Hence, self-management control rests with the person and is often shared with peers. It challenges the expert view of knowledge exchange/transfer. It involves health-care teams with relevant skills and resources to support and assist, enabling them to interact more productively with patients and each other. This shared responsibility with health professionals, based on principles of genuine collaboration, involves understanding and respecting individuals' personal and cultural beliefs, wishes and circumstances and those of family, collaborative identification of problems and goals, negotiated care plans and active follow-up (Whitby 2003).

Taylor (1979) identifies a number of issues in helping people who are similar to a self-management model by seeing them as 'predicaments'. They highlight that the person needs to recognise that there is a problem, that they need help to overcome the problem, that they bear primary responsibility for change, that it is worthwhile trying to change behaviour and that change is supported by modifying bio-psychosocial factors with the help of help-givers who can be professional, informal supports and/or family/carers.

Central to self-management is the notion of rights and responsibilities and how these are shared. These, and the ability to exercise control by the person, are tempered by levels of access to information and resources and by social determinants of health, that is the social, economic, political and cultural structures that perpetuate health inequity (Lynch *et al.* 1997; Diderichsen *et al.* 2001; Burchardt 2003; Wilkinson & Marmot 2003; Hetzel *et al.* 2004).

Self-efficacy and behaviour change

Self-management requires the person to hold the belief that they can effectively self-manage their condition and to have improved self-efficacy or confidence in their ability to self-care, which involves cognitive, perceptual, behavioural and lifestyle changes. There is a large amount of literature that links a number of issues to self-care and self-care enhancement through change. These are discussed below.

Self-efficacy, according to Bandura, can be defined as the confidence one has in one's ability to perform a specific behaviour or to change a specific cognition. Bandura proposed that this is a major determinant of patients' health behaviours, that the strength of belief in one's capability, not necessarily 'true' capability, is a good predictor of future motivation and behaviours (Bandura 1977; Bandura *et al.* 1977). Baseline self-efficacy and changes in self-efficacy have been shown to be associated with future health status and health behaviours in people with chronic diseases (Lorig *et al.* 2001). There needs to be a thorough assessment of self-efficacy to understand how this might be present and be interpreted differently by people from different cultural backgrounds.

Marlatt and Gordon (1985) have articulated steps for relapse prevention involving cue exposure, role-playing risk situations and challenging beliefs such as the abstinence violation effect. Most action plans and symptom action plans are based on such premises. Janis and Mann (1977) developed the decisional balance model to explain how the person undertakes problem-solving by considering the pros and cons of changing behaviour in a structured approach.

Prochaska and DiClemente (1983) described the process of change in their transtheoretical model which has been widely referred to. Many projects have found that the most important determinant for successful behaviour change is the state of readiness of the individual to embrace change. This is just as important for service providers and services. Change is often perceived as a process of 'plugging away' and waiting for the process to mature (Orpin & Frendin 2003). This model has been widely criticised because it is largely limited to describing the process rather than explaining how change occurs. It offers little for those individuals, groups and systems that continue to be pre-contemplators, either by choice or because they feel disempowered to contemplate a change in their circumstances because of psychosocial factors. Motivational interviewing (Miller 1980; Miller & Rollnick 1991) is a client-centred counselling style for eliciting behaviour change by helping clients to explore and resolve ambivalence to change. It is also focused and goal directed.

Central to self-efficacy is the ability to identify issues, set goals and build commitment to actions, within the context of a problem-solving approach. These cognitive and behavioural interventions have been found to be as effective as taking tricyclic anti-depressants and more effective than selective serotonin reuptake inhibitors (SSRIs) for improving outcomes for people with mild depression. The best outcomes have also been achieved when a good therapeutic alliance is formed between the health-care professional and the patient, over a long period of treatment (Ellis & Smith 2002). In general, meta-analysis of research has found this approach to be positively correlated with overall health outcomes (Penley *et al.* 2002).

Resilience

An aspect of self-care is the innate and immediate responses we use for self-preservation. Self-preservation responses are inherent to the notion of resilience, which is now no longer perceived as something special but rather something that most people have, and all are able to develop given the right supports to do so (Deveson 2003). Resilience is akin to protective factors, and relies on factors inherent in the individual and those existing resources of the community. Hence, solutions can potentially be found beyond the health-care system.

The person's reaction to the development of a chronic condition also needs to be understood. To date in the literature, there has not been a great deal of focus on the adaptation required when a person develops a chronic condition. There is little doubt that the life crisis literature has a great deal of information about adaptation to chronic diseases by children and adults and the fact that if this adaptation does not occur, poor health outcomes result (Riessman & Carroll 1995; Deveson 2003).

Resilience is closely linked to the concept of predicaments and how each person interprets his or her experience of chronic illness within his or her environment. Taylor (1979) reminds us that 'no matter how much we learn about mechanisms within the body, the interface between the individual and the environment is personal and determined by attitudes and experience' (p. 1010). Therefore, the differential susceptibility to illness behaviour and disease can only be understood by studying the role of predicaments, the 'complex of psychosocial ramifications, contacts, meanings, and ascriptions which bear upon the individual' (p. 1009). Although a person may be resilient regardless of his/her socio-economic status, the social determinants of health inequity bear heavily on populations where poverty, lack of employment and educational opportunities and other social determinants are prominent. These populations tend to have the worst health outcomes. Promoting and supporting resilience by addressing such inequities would be an important component of the chronic disease strategy. Likewise, encouraging health workers to see and acknowledge their patients' strengths and resilience in spite of potentially longstanding chronic illness and complex and insidious psychosocial pressures may not only empower the worker but also the patient.

Compliance and adherence

Self-management includes the actions that people take in relation to the advice given by health professionals. Patient adherence or compliance to prescribed treatment has been recognised as a major problem in achieving optimal outcomes in chronic illness care (Vermeire *et al.* 2001). *Compliance* has been defined as 'the extent to which a person's behaviour, in terms of taking medications, following diets, executing lifestyle changes coincided with medical or health advice'. Non-compliance with medication makes a substantial contribution to poor health outcomes (Thorne *et al.* 2000) though the reasons for this are poorly understood. Compliance can be improved by the delivery method of educational interventions. For example, there is evidence that self-help interventions have only a small impact and effect on behaviour change leading to improved health. However, using the example of smokers wishing to quit, material tailored for individuals have been shown to be more effective (Lancaster & Stead 2002).

Compliance fits well with an acute illness. However, the person with a chronic condition may view his or her situation differently and is likely to be viewed differently by health professionals. The word 'compliance' has moral connotations and implies that non-compliance is associated with psychological problems. The word 'concordance' has been proposed because it conveys the idea that the patient decides whether what is asked of him or her matches his or her own beliefs and attitudes. The term 'adherence' has gained in acceptance because it combines the broader notions of concordance, cooperation and partnership (Vermeire *et al.* 2001).

Patient-centred care

The concept of 'patient-centred care' has gained attention over the last three decades as an alternative to what was seen as the traditional didactic 'medical model' approach to doctor–patient interactions. This concept or process was seen as a way of improving adherence to recommended medical advice to improve health outcomes. Bauman *et al.* (2003) describe patient-centred care as the sharing of the management of an illness between patient and doctor using three elements: (a) communication, (b) partnerships and (c) a focus beyond specific conditions, on health promotion and healthy lifestyles. Stewart (2001) defines patient-centred care from the patient's perspective as 'care which (a) explores the patient's main reason for the visit, concerns and need for information; (b) seeks an integrated understanding of the patient's world – that is, their whole person, emotional needs, life issues; (c) finds common ground on what the problem is and mutually agrees on management; (d) enhances prevention and health promotion; and (e) enhances the continuing relationship between the doctor and the patient.' Bauman *et al.* (2003) note the increasing evidence for the effectiveness of patient-centred approaches. The authors also include self-management training as part of patient-centred care along with goal setting, written management plans and regular follow-ups.

Patient activation

In the United States, patient activation is a term which describes similar concepts as self-management (Hibbard *et al.* 2004). Patient activation is stated to be the outcome of the implementation of the Chronic Care Model (Wagner *et al.* 2001). The idea of patient activation is the assumption that patients are likely to make good decisions if they are informed and feel confident that they can take care of themselves (Von Korff *et al.* 1998; Lorig *et al.* 1999). Activation is seen as a process that a person with a chronic condition goes through. It consists of the knowledge, skill and confidence for self-management of chronic conditions and develops in four stages: (a) believing that the patient's role is important; (b) having the confidence and knowledge necessary to take action; (c) actually taking action to maintain and improve one's health; and (d) staying on the course even under stress (Hibbard *et al.* 2004). The concept has been developed into a questionnaire (the Patient Activation Measure) with 22 items based around the four domains described above. It has been validated in the United States and the United Kingdom and has been shown to be predictive of health-care status, utilisation and health behaviours (Hibbard *et al.* 2004; Ellins *et al.* 2005).

The role of support

Empirically, social support has been linked to better health outcomes (Murray *et al.* 2006). Social support has been described by Cobb (1976) as the provision of information that they are cared for and loved, that they belong to a network of mutual obligation and that they are esteemed and valued. Weiss (1973) established that this information is provided by five categories of relationships which provide intimacy, the opportunity to exercise nurturing behaviour, a sense of social integration, reassurance of worth and practical assistance. Many relationships are adversely affected by the onset of symptomatic chronic diseases or conditions.

Both patients and carers need to learn how to maintain their close supportive relationships and thereby their sense of support. The 'significant others' are also central to achieving the health outcomes required for people with chronic diseases. People with chronic conditions often deal with their health problems outside the health-care system, using their own informal resources, often with the help of family and friends, informal and formal carers and a range of community resources and support networks not directly linked with health services. Therefore, this support needs to be acknowledged and utilised effectively as part of any plan of self-management support (Australian Bureau of Statistics 2003).

Validity and measurability of self-management

The construct validity of self-management is a significant issue. Existing reviews and meta-analyses of self-management research have been problematic and are often criticised because of the diversity of studies and health conditions, varied research methods and lack of clarity about what is being measured (Warsi *et al.* 2004). Camp Quality for children with serious illnesses such as malignancy is an example. To conduct a randomised controlled trial on such a programme would seem to be redundant. This is because there needs to be greater clarity about 'what' is being measured. Randomised controlled trials (RCTs) have been proposed as the most effective method of evaluating health-care treatments and interventions (Altman 1996).

However, ethnic minorities (Hussain-Gambles *et al.* 2004), people who have mental illness and other vulnerable groups have often been subject to exclusion from RCTs, with little justification. The effect this has on RCT results and knowledge, generally about the area being investigated in self-management research, is unclear. Arguably, their exclusion potentially limits the scope of knowledge and learning, misses important aspects and variables and limits what is actually being measured in the first place. In addition to this, the development of reliable and valid scales to rate elements of shared decision-making in clinical encounters has also been proposed (Fenton 2003).

It is not known whether generic models of self-management are more or less effective than interventions developed for specific conditions or whether a generic model has equal effectiveness with a range of chronic conditions. Emerging research suggests that there are differences that need more thorough investigation (Gibson *et al.* 2004; Newman *et al.* 2004). For example, a meta-analysis by Warsi *et al.* (2004) suggests that self-management programmes are effective for asthma and diabetes but not for arthritis, though this review has been criticised for its lack of rigour.

Likewise, self-management courses such as those using the Stanford group model have produced varied results with various conditions with little under-standing of exactly which elements of the courses are effective in improving which outcomes, whether some outcomes should have greater priority than oth-ers, to what extent self-management interventions address health inequalities (income, education, literacy, gender, culture, etc.) and which population groups are more successful or less so. The overall high participant satisfaction has often been counterbalanced by little change in pain level and visits to doctors. Sustainability of self-management gains once the person ceases involvement in courses has also been an issue of concern. Very little is understood about the process generally.

'There is no health without mental health'

There is also a need to recognise that self-management is difficult for any individual to acquire and sustain and that the role exerted by mental illnesses and emotional well-being is generally a little researched or understood area (Chapman *et al.* 2005). This is clearly linked to how successful the person is at self-managing and how the person's motivation to self-manage is supported by others in the longer term. Therefore, self-management must incorporate an understanding of how mental health interacts with the physical health of the person in both causal and consequential ways. WHO predictions are that by the year 2020, depressive disorders will be second only to heart disease in the global burden of disease (Murray & Lopez. 1996). Chapman *et al.* (2005) demonstrate that depression shares a fundamental relationship with physical illness:

- Depression may occur in up to 50% of people with asthma.
- Depression and anxiety are the most commonly reported concerns for people with arthritis.
- People with depression are much more likely to develop coronary artery disease.
- Depression is also predictive of stroke and myocardial infarction (four times more likely than those with no history of depression), with depression highly likely to develop as a consequence of these conditions.
- Research suggests strong links with cancer and mental illness, either via risk factors (e.g. smoking) and their consequences or as a direct consequence of the impact of cancer and its treatment.
- Depression is twice as prevalent amongst people with diabetes as among those without diabetes.
- There is a significant relationship between obesity and depression among women.
- Depression is related to mortality in cardiovascular disease.

These points are confirmed by the Busselton study in Western Australia that found people with mental illness had 2.5 times the death rate from all major physical health conditions than people without mental illness (Coghlan *et al.* 2001). Lifestyle risk factors such as high rates of smoking, poor diet and low physical activity levels and their consequences, problems with accessing primary care providers and problems with early detection and treatment of physical conditions may all be contributing factors.

Sustainability

Definitions of self-management imply ongoing self-care beyond the initial self-management education that arises from contact with professional and informal supports. However, sustainability of gains from existing programmes and strategies is uncertain. Some studies with people with diabetes have found that improvements decline with time (Norris *et al.* 2001). Problems with sustainability have been noted by several studies with participants rarely initiating follow-up and motivation declining post course without it. A structured and regular review has been found to be effective in improving the process of care (Renders *et al.* 2000) as have interventions that have included a combination of reminders, self-monitoring, reinforcement, counselling, family therapy and other forms of supervision, though these improvements are not large (Haynes *et al.* 2002).

Larger issues of sustainability involve ensuring agencies' commitment to continuing and enhancing their programmes into the future and providing them with the incentives to do so. Using the diabetes example, effective delivery system design has had a proven impact on outcomes for patients (Sperl-Hillen *et al.* 2004). There is also the potential problem of perceiving accountability for outcomes resting entirely with the individual who could then be blamed for the failure to self-manage. Hence, sustainability is also about ensuring quality and accountability into the future. This could be managed by developing structured education, training and accreditation mechanisms across the health sector as well as developing and implementing systemic monitoring processes that support the patient and the significant others and that assist the health professional to monitor and not lose heart or become complacent over the long haul.

Self-management support

The professional assists the person with a range of tasks that will promote effective self-management based on the person's goals, wishes and capacities by addressing and encouraging client participation in key skills of problem-solving, decision-making and confidence-building. This is achieved by addressing central tasks regarding role, emotional management and medically related tasks using a client-centred holistic approach that builds on the clients' capacity, strengths, resilience and dignity.

In the United States, the emphasis has been on the health professionals' role in self-management support. Bodenheimer *et al.* (2005) start from the position of self management support before defining self-management. They define self-management support as 'the assistance caregivers give patients to encourage daily decisions that improve health-related behaviors and clinical outcomes. Self-management support includes a portfolio of techniques and tools that help patients choose healthy behaviors. But it also encompasses a fundamental transformation of the patient-caregiver relationship into a collaborative partnership' (p. 5).

The Institute of Medicine defines self-management support as the systematic provision of information and skills, that is, providing evidence-based information, teaching disease-specific skills, supporting healthy behaviours, developing problem-solving skills, helping the person manage the emotional impact of the condition, providing active follow-up and active participation by the person with the condition in his or her own care.

Alternative definitions of self-management

In the United Kingdom, the NHS has adopted self-care as the term to encompass self-management. 'Self care is all about individuals taking responsibility for their own health and well-being. This includes staying fit and healthy, both physically and mentally; taking action to prevent illness and accidents; the better use of medicines; treatment of minor ailments and better care of long term conditions' (Department of Health 2006). The NHS policy document then adopts the Rethink definition of self-management as 'whatever we do to make the most of our lives by coping with difficulties and making the most of what we have' (Department of Health 2006). Elsewhere, self-care is defined as the actions individuals take to lead a healthy lifestyle, to meet their social, emotional and psychological needs; to care for their long-term condition; and to prevent further illness or accidents (Barlow *et al*. 2002).

Australian conceptualisations of self-management

The Council of Australian Governments identified the prevention and management of chronic conditions as a national priority in 1995 (COAG Task Force on Health and Community Services 1995) and funded the national coordinated care trials to test models of delivering improved care within existing costs. SA Health-Plus was the largest of the national trials and aimed to improve self-management as one of its conceptual approaches to improving chronic care. The controlled trial enrolled 4500 participants (3100 intervention patients) in eight projects. One of the key outcomes of the trial was based on a mid-trial review with service coordinators who were trained to use behavioural methods of problem definition and goal setting to assist patients with self-management. They reported that although the overall model of care planning and behavioural change approaches were successful, they were providing care and coordination based more on a patient's capacity for self-management rather than on his or her illness severity or complexity. This led to the development of the Partners in Health programme by the Flinders Human Behaviour and Health Research Unit (FHBHRU), which aimed to devise an objective way to assess self-management. This programme was based on a literature review, which found that there was no structured clinician-administered process to assess a patient's self-management and no questionnaires to assess self-management (Battersby *et al*. 2003).

The literature review identified a definition of self-management provided by the Center for the Advancement of Health and Center for Health Studies Group Health Cooperative of Puget Sound (1996), which was endorsed by a series of patient and health professional focus groups: self-management 'involves (the person with the chronic condition) engaging in activities that protect and promote health, monitoring and managing the symptoms and signs of illness, managing the impact of illness on functioning, emotions and interpersonal relationships and adhering to treatment regimes'. These elements (the three tasks of disease, role and emotional management) are similarly defined by Lorig and Holman (2003b) and Corbin and Strauss (1988).

Based on this definition, the FHBHRU identified six principles of self-management. These principles described the six core tasks for individuals with chronic conditions to maximise their self-management capacity. From these six principles, a patient rated self-assessment of self-management was created using an 11-item Likert scale (Partners in Health scale). This was complemented by the clinician's motivational interview using the same 11 items expanded with open-ended questions (Cue and Response [C&R] interview). Combined with the Problem and Goal Assessment (Battersby *et al.* 2001) these three components led to the development of what has become known as the Flinders model care plan.

What was also clear from the HealthPlus trial was the fact that to ensure that a population of 3100 patients adhered as best as possible to evidence-based care guidelines, clinicians had to be provided with a systematic and systemic means by which self-management and medical management could be firstly integrated and secondly monitored within the real world of everyday practice. This meant that monitoring had to be the measurement of health outcomes to achieve evidence-based medicine (EBM) goals and self-management by the measurement of patient-defined problems and goals in their own terms. And both needed to be done concurrently, longitudinally and in an integrated way. To achieve this, the EBM guidelines were converted into an operationalised format 'the care plan generator', which outlined the tasks that needed to be done over the next 12 months to medically manage and monitor each chronic condition as well as the requirements to achieve risk factor reduction. The self-management component then addressed problems and goals including strategies to deal with symptom monitoring and symptom-action plans, as well as the achievement of personal goals. A service coordinator facilitated this process, resulting in an integrated care plan for each patient that was signed by the patient (and or carer), the service coordinator and the medical practitioner responsible. This ensured a patient-centred care planning process, the recording and monitoring of both EBM care and patient problems and goal (P&G) achievement. In effect, both, patients and health professionals had symbolically and actually changed roles by making what is usually an implicit contract into a conscious and committed reality. This is shown figuratively in Figures 5.2 and 5.3.

Impact of the Flinders model
Research and Policy Development

Since 2000, the FHBHRU has conducted a series of projects for the Commonwealth Department of Health and Ageing including a clinician self-management education module for the national Sharing Health Care Demonstration projects and the development of the self-management action plan for the National Chronic Disease Strategy. In 2006, the Council of Australian Governments established the Australian Better Health Initiative (ABHI) to address the emerging crisis in chronic conditions. A core element of the initiative is the education of the future (Pols & Battersby 2006) and current Australian workforce in self-management support. FHBHRU was contracted to develop a national curriculum for self-management support for all undergraduate and professional entry courses across Australia for nursing, allied health and medical professions. A key aspect of this project was

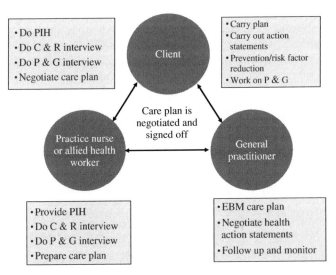

Figure 5.2   The Flinders Model: a systemic approach.

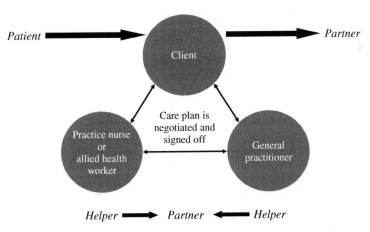

Figure 5.3   The Flinders Model: a patient-centred partnership approach.

to develop an agreed definition and common terminology for self-management (Battersby *et al*. 2007).

Self-management support is defined as

The process of providing multi-level resources in health-care systems (and the community) to facilitate a person's self-management. It includes the social, physical and emotional support given by health professionals, significant others and/or carers and other supports to assist a person in managing their chronic condition. Self-management support is what health professionals and the health system do to assist the person with a chronic condition to manage their condition(s). It includes a health system that provides ready access to appropriate systems of self-management support that are: Evidence-based and adequately resourced with staff who are adequately trained, culturally sensitive to the person's needs and who support the belief in the person's ability to learn self-management skills.

The corresponding project to determine the training needs of the Australian primary care workforce in prevention and self-management of chronic conditions has also involved a national consultation and final workshop that endorsed the definitions developed as part of the curriculum project.

Clinical trials

There have been several generic and disease-specific projects using the Flinders model. The model's tools provide a generic and accessible means of assessing clients' self-management ability that leads directly to the development of a multidisciplinary care plan. The Stanford group-based model and the Flinders individual-based models are complementary approaches to chronic condition self-management, which have been used effectively with those considered at most disadvantage and risk within the community (Lawn *et al.* 2007; Harvey *et al.* 2008). In addition, the Flinders self-management model incorporates patient-centred self-management education complemented by a focus on comprehensive worker education through workforce training and clinical skills improvement that assists them to effectively support self-management by patients.

Health professional education and training

Effective education of and support to the workforce have been critical as part of these approaches, recognising the fact that overcoming negative workforce culture, attitudes and beliefs about patients is central to the process of effective engagement in self-management. Supporting the health workforce to develop skills to communicate effectively with patients in a person-centred way to support behaviour change and to understand the impact of health systems on patients is pivotal to the success of any self-management programme. This has been confirmed as part of a national survey of the skills and information needed by the Australian primary health-care workforce and audit of training organisations, and recommendations arising from this study (Battersby *et al.* 2008).

FHBHRU has used this conceptualisation of self-management to develop a 2-day training programme in self-management support, which has been provided to over 4000 health professionals across Australia, New Zealand, the United States and Canada. Several research studies have used the Flinders model as part of the intervention, demonstrating improved self-management, clinical and service utilisation outcomes (Harvey 2001; Lawn *et al.* 2007). In this way, a holistic definition of self-management has provided the foundation for a semi-structured clinical method that enables the patient to be included collaboratively in their own care. This clinician-based interview provides an inherent motivational framework to guide behaviour change and improve adherence to the agreed care plan. This approach has within it the core elements of self-care, patient-centred care, empowerment and patient engagement.

Education in the Flinders model of self-management is formalised with an online-based postgraduate certificate and diploma offered through Flinders University and a dedicated workforce development programme that supports several projects and programmes throughout South Australia and other states.

Conclusions: the future for chronic condition self-management

The conceptualisation of chronic condition self-management (CCSM) is still at a rather early stage of our empirical knowledge and understanding. Medical practice in the developed world suffers from the accident of history that the acute care model was adopted because of the needs of war and infectious diseases because of the acute care that was demanded by those circumstances. This was cemented because of the needs for education and training of the health-care workforce where the large hospital became the focus for such learning. In contrast, the CCSM approach results in patient-driven consultations initiated by patient demand rather than the need and allocation of health-care resources that contrasts with the strategies that are required if the epidemic of the burden of diseases in the ageing population is to be contained within the bounds of reasonable expenditures.

There remains a major need for an informed community debate about the responsibility that has to be accepted by all citizens for their own self-management and preventative health care. Education of the health-care workforce is a slow process that takes 5–10 years to effect change if universities implement the required changes. These institutions are also slow to change. Culturally there is much misinformation available to patients. Much of this information is pushed by marketing and is not evidence-based. There are also cultural issues for policymakers with the three related epidemics of obesity, sedentary and passive behaviour and type 2 diabetes that are also pertinent to concepts of self-management. Should there be universal exercise in the form of a sports curriculum and preventative health-care curriculum within the education system and support for exercise-based healthy diet and lifestyle community programmes for all people so that 'the activated patient' can more readily become a reality rather than a small minority of the population?

For now, however, the FHBHRU continues to work with patients, policymakers, educationists and clinicians to implement what is known and to try to add to the body of knowledge in this area.

References

Alcoholics Anonymous. (2007) *The Big Book Online*, 4th edition, from http://www.aa.org/bigbookonline/ (accessed in 2007).

Altman, D. (1996) Better reporting of randomised controlled trials: the consort statement. *British Medical Journal* 313: 570–571.

American Diabetes Association. *DiabetesPro Professional Resources*. Professional Meetings/Education. Retrieved 11 January 2008, from http://professional.diabetes. org/Meetings_GeneralList.aspx.

Anderson, R.M., Funnell, M.M., Butler, P.M., Arnold, M.S., Fitzgerald, J.T., Feste, C.C. (1995) Patient empowerment: results of a randomized controlled trial. *Diabetes Care* 18(7): 943–949.

Australian Bureau of Statistics. (2003) *Disability, Ageing and Carers, Australia: Summary of Findings. CAT 4430.0.* Retrieved 4 February 2005, from http://www.abs.gov.au/ Ausstats/abs@.nsf/0/c258c88a7aa5a87eca2568a9001393e8?opendocument.

Bandura, A. (1977) Self-efficacy: toward a unifying theory of behavioral change. *Psychological Review* 84(2): 191–215.

Bandura, A., Adams, N., Beyer, J. (1977) Cognitive processes mediating behavioral change. *Journal of Personality and Social Psychology* 35: 125–139.

Barlow, J., Wright, C., Sheasby, J., Turner, A., Hainsworth, J. (2002) Self-management approaches for people with chronic conditions: a review. *Patient Education and Counseling* 48(2): 177–187.

Battersby, M.W. (2006) A risk worth taking. *Chronic Illness* 2(4): 265–269.

Battersby, M.W., Ask, A., Reece, M.M., Markwick, M.J., Collins, J.P. (2001) A case study using the "problems and goals approach" in a coordinated care trial: SA HealthPlus. *Australian Journal of Primary Health* 7(3): 45–48.

Battersby, M., Ask, A., Reece, M., Markwick, M., Collins, J. (2003) The partners in health scale: the development and psychometric properties of a generic assessment scale for chronic condition self-management. *Australian Journal of Primary Health* 9(2–3): 41–52.

Battersby, M., Lawn, S., Reed, R. *et al.* (2007) *The Development of a Framework to Guide the Integration of Chronic Disease Self-management into Undergraduate Curricula.* Commonwealth Department of Health and Ageing: Adelaide.

Battersby, M.W., Lawn, S., Wells, L. *et al.* (2008, in submission) *An Audit of the Training and Information Needs of the Australian Primary Health Care Workforce.* Commonwealth Department of Health and Ageing: Adelaide.

Bauman, A.E., Fardy, H.J., Harris, P.G. (2003) Getting it right: why bother with patient-centred care? *Medical Journal of Australia* 179: 253–256.

Benyshek, D.C. (2005) Type 2 diabetes and fetal origins: the promise of prevention programs focusing on prenatal health in high prevalence Native American communities. *Society for Applied Anthropology* 64(2): 192–200.

Bodenheimer, T., McGregor, K., Shafiri, C. (2005) *California Health Report: Helping Patients Manage their Chronic Conditions.*

Brooks, M. (2002) *Sharing the Journey.* New Paradigm Press: North Fitzroy.

Burchardt, T. (2003) *Being and Becoming: Social Exclusion and the Onset of Disability.* Case Report 21. ESRC Centre for Analysis of Social Exclusion/London School of Economics: London.

Caplan, G. (1964). *Principles of Preventative Psychiatry.* Basic Books Inc.: New York, pp. 38–54.

Center for the Advancement of Health and Center for Health Studies Group Health Cooperative of Puget Sound. (1996) *An Indexed Bibliography on Self-management for People with Chronic Disease.* Center for the Advancement of Health: Washington, DC.

Chapman, D., Perry, G., Strine, T.W. (2005) The vital link between chronic disease and depressive disorders. *Preventing Chronic Disease, Public Health Research, Practice and Policy* **2**(1–10).

COAG Task Force on Health and Community Services. (1995) *Health and Community Services: Meeting People's Needs Better – A Discussion Paper*. Commonwealth Department of Human Services and Health: Canberra.

Cobb, S. (1976) Social support as a moderator of life stresses. *Psychosomatic Medicine* **38**: 300–314.

Coghlan, R., Lawrence, D., Holman, C., Jablensky, A. (2001) *Duty of Care: Physical Health in People with Mental Illness*. Technical Report. Centre for Health Services Research, School of Population Health, The University of Western Australia: Perth.

Connors, C. (2005) Compliance – Let's get Real! Part 1. *The Chronicle* **7**(6): 1–3.

Corben, S., Rosen, R. (2005) *Self-management for Long-term Conditions: Patients' Perspectives on the Way Ahead*. King's Fund: London.

Corbin, J.M., Strauss, A. (1988) *Unending Work and Care: Managing Chronic Illness at Home*. Jossey-Bass Inc.: San Francisco, CA.

Creer, T., Christian, W. (1976) *Chronically Ill and Handicapped Children*. Research Press: Champaign, IL.

Davidson, L. (2004) *Recovery in Serious Mental Illness: Paradigm Shift or Shibboleth? Keynote Address, Recovery: Challenging the Paradigm*. 6th Biennial VICSERV Mental Health Conference, Melbourne.

Department of Health. (2006) *Supporting People with Long Term Conditions to Self Care – A Guide to Developing Local Strategies and Good Practice*. NHS: Adelaide.

Deveson, A. (2003) *Resilience*. Allen & Unwin: Crows Nest.

Diderichsen, F., Evans, T., Whitehead, M. (2001) The social bias of disparities in health. In: Evans, T., Whitehead, M., Diderichsen, F., Buyia, A., Wirth, M. (eds) *Challenging Inequalities in Health*. Oxford University Press: Oxford, pp. 13–23.

Drew, L. (1987) Beyond the disease concept of addition: towards integration of the moral and scientific perspectives. *Australian Drug and Alcohol Review* **6**: 45–48.

Ellins, J., Coulter, A.; Picker Institute Europe. (2005) *How Engaged Are People in Their Healthcare?: Findings of a National Telephone Survey*. The Health Foundation.

Ellis, P.M., Smith, D.A. (2002) Treating depression: the beyondblue guidelines for treating depression in primary care. *Medical Journal of Australia* **176** (Suppl 10): S77–S83.

Farrell, C. (2004) *Patient and Public Involvement in Health: The Evidence for Policy Implementation*. Department of Health: London.

Fenton, W.S. (2003) Editorial: shared decision making: a model for the physician-patient relationship in the 21st century? *Acta Psychiatrica Scandinavia* **107**: 401–402.

Funnell, M.M., Anderson, R.M. (2004) Empowerment and self-management of diabetes. *Clinical Diabetes* **22**(3): 123–127.

Funnell, M., Anderson, R.M., Arnold, M. *et al.* (1991) Empowerment: an idea whose time has come in diabetes education. *The Diabetes Educator* **17**(1): 37–41.

Gibson, P., Coughlan, J., Wilson, A. *et al.* (2004) Self-management education and regular practitioner review for adults with asthma. *Cochrane Database of Systematic Reviews* Issue 4: Art. No: CD001117.

Golan, N. (1974) Crisis theory. In: Turner, F. (ed.) *Social Work Treatment: Interlocking Theoretical Approaches*. Free Press: New York, pp. 296–340.

Gunderson, E., Rahe, R.E. (1974) *Life Events and Illness*. Thomas: Springfield, IL.

Hamman, J., Leucht, S., Kissling, W. (2003) Shared decision making in psychiatry. *Acta Psychiatrica Scandinavica* **107**: 403–409.

Harvey, P.W. (2001) The impact of coordinated care: Eyre region, South Australia 1997–1999. *Australian Journal of Rural Health* **9**(2): 70–74.

Harvey, P.W., Petkov, J.N., Misan, G. *et al.* (2008) Self-management support and training for patients with chronic and complex conditions improves health-related behaviour and health outcomes. *Australian Health Review* **32**(2): 330–338.

Haynes, R., McDonald, H., Garg, A., Montague, P. (2002) Interventions for helping patients to follow prescriptions for medications. *Cochrane Database of Systematic Reviews* Issue 2: Art. No.: CD000011. DOI: 10.1002/14651858.CD000011.

Hetzel, D., Page, A., Glover, J., Tennant, S. (2004) *Inequality in South Australia: Key Determinants of Wellbeing, The Evidence*, Vol. 1. Department of Health: Adelaide, p. 112.

Hibbard, J., Sockard, J., Mahoney, E.R., Tusler, M. (2004) Development of the Patient Activation Measure (PAM): conceptualizing and measuring activation in patients and consumers. *Health Services Research* **39**: 1005–1026.

Horne, R., Weinman, J. (1999) Patient's beliefs about prescribed medicines and their role in adherence to treatment. *Clinical Journal of Psychosomatic Research* **47**: 555–567.

Hussain-Gambles, M., Atkin, K., Leese, B. (2004) Why ethnic minority groups are under-represented in clinical trials: a review of the literature. *Health and Social Care in the Community* **12**(5): 382–388.

Ignatieff, M. (1994) *The Needs of Strangers*. Vintage: London.

Janis, I., Mann, L. (1977) *Decision Making: A Psychological Analysis of Conflict, Choice, and Commitment*. Free Press: New York.

Lancaster, T., Stead, L. (2002) Self-help interventions for smoking cessation. *The Cochrane Database of Systematic Reviews* Issue 3: Art. No.: CD001118. DOI: 10.1002/14651858.CD001118.

Lawn, S., Battersby, M., Pols, R.G., Lawrence, J., Parry, T., Urukalo, M. (2007) The mental health expert patient: findings from a pilot study of a generic chronic condition self-management programme for people with mental illness. *International Journal of Social Psychiatry* **53**(1): 63–74.

Lorig, K. (1993) Self-management of chronic illness: a model for the future (self care and older adults). *Generations* **17**(3): 11–14.

Lorig, K., Holman, H. (2003a) Self-management Education: Context, Definition and Outcomes and Mechanisms. *First Chronic Disease Self-Management Conference*, Sydney.

Lorig, K.R., Holman, H.R. (2003b) Self-management education: history, definition, outcomes, and mechanisms. *Annals of Behavioral Medicine* **26**(1): 1–7.

Lorig, K., Ritter, P., Stewart, A. *et al.* (2001) Chronic disease self-management program: 2-year health status and health care utilization outcomes. *Medical Care* **39**(11): 1217–1223.

Lorig, K., Sobel, D., Stewart, A. *et al.* (1999) Evidence suggesting that a chronic disease self-management program can improve health status while reducing hospitalization: a randomized trial. *Medical Care* **37**(1): 5–14.

Lynch, J., Kaplan, G., Shema, S. (1997) Cumulative impact of sustained economic hardship on physical, cognitive, psychological and social functioning. *Massachusetts Medical Society* **337**(26): 1889–1895.

Marlatt, G., Gordon, J. (1985) *Relapse Prevention*. The Guilford Press: New York.

Miller, W. (1980) The addictive behaviours. In: Miller, W. (ed.) *The Addictive Behaviours: Treatment of Alcoholism, Drug Abuse, Smoking, And Obesity*, Chapter 1. Pergamon Press: Oxford, pp. 3–10.

Miller, W. (1990) Spirituality: the silent dimension in addiction research. The 1990 Leonard Ball oration. *Drug and Alcohol Review* 9: 259–266.

Miller, W.R., Rollnick, S. (1991) *Motivational Interviewing Preparing People to Change Addictive Behavior*. The Guilford Press: New York.

Murray, E., Burns, J., See Tai, S., Lai, R., Nazareth, I. (2006) Interactive health communication applications for people with chronic disease. *The Cochrane Database of Systematic Reviews* Issue 4.

Murray, C., Lopez, A. (eds) (1996) *The Global Burden of Disease*. Harvard University Press: Harvard.

Newbould, J., Taylor, D., Bury, M. (2006) Lay-led self-management in chronic illness: a review of the evidence. *Chronic Illness* 2(4): 249–261.

Newman, S., Steed, L., Mulligan, K. (2004) Self-management interventions for chronic illness. *The Lancet* **364**: 1523–1537.

Norris, S., Engelgau, M., Narayan, K. (2001) Effectiveness of self-management training in type 2 diabetes: a systematic review of randomized controlled trails. *Diabetes Care* **24**: 561–587.

Orpin, P., Frendin, S. (2003) A time for every purpose – patience is a virtue in effecting change. *Guiding Us Forward: National Chronic Condition Self-Management Conference*. Australian Government Department of Health & Ageing: Melbourne.

Penley, J.A., Tomaka, J., Wiebe, J.S. (2002) The association of coping to physical and psychological health outcomes: a meta-analytic review. *Journal of Behavioral Medicine* **25**(6): 551–603.

Pepper, S. (2002) *Towards Recovery*, Vol. 1. New Paradigm Press: North Fitzroy.

Pols, R.G., Battersby, M.W. (2006) Chronic condition self-management: is there a need for a specific curriculum for medical students? *Medical Education* **40**: 719–721.

Prochaska, J., DiClemente, C. (1983) Stages and processes of self-change of smoking: towards an integrated model of change. *Journal of Consulting and Clinical Psychology* **51**: 390–395.

Renders, C., Valk, G., Griffin, S., Wagner, E.H., van Eijjk, J.T., Assendelft, W.J. (2000) Interventions to improve the management of diabetes mellitus in primary care, outpatient and community settings. *The Cochrane Database of Systematic Reviews* Issue 4: Art. No.: CD001481. DOI: 10.1002/14651858.CD001481.

Riessman, F., Carroll, D. (1995) *Redefining Self-Help: Policy and Practice*. Jossey-Bass Publishers: San Francisco, CA.

Rogers, A. (2006) Damned by faint praise? *Chronic Illness* 2: 262–264.

Roter, D.L., Hall, J.A., Merisca, R., Nordstrom, B., Cretin, D., Svarstad, B. (1998) Effectiveness of interventions to improve patient compliance: a meta-analysis. *Medical Care* **36**(8): 1138–1161.

Shaw, J., Baker, M. (2004) "Expert patient"– dream or nightmare? *British Medical Journal* **328**(7442): 723–724.

Shulman, A. (1992) *The Skills of Helping: Individuals, Families and Groups*. F. E. Peacock Publishing Company: Itasca, IL.

Sperl-Hillen, J.M., Solberg, L.I., Hroseikoski, M.C., Crain, A.L., Engebretson, K.I., O'Connor, P.J. (2004) Do all components of the chronic care model contribute equally to quality improvement? *Joint Commission Journal on Quality and Safety* **30**(6): 303–309.

Stewart, M. (2001) Towards a global definition of patient centred care. *British Medical Journal* **322**(7284): 444–445.

Taylor, D.C. (1979) The components of sickness: diseases, illnesses, and predicaments. *The Lancet* **10**: 1008–1010.

Thorne, S., Ternulf Nyhlin, K., Paterson, B. (2000) Attitudes towards patient expertise in chronic illness. *International Journal of Nursing Studies* **37**: 303–311.

Vermeire, E., Hearnshaw, H., Van Royen, P., Denekens, J. (2001) Patient adherence to treatment: three decades of research. A comprehensive review. *Journal of Clinical Pharmacy and Therapeutics* **26**: 331–342.

Von Korff, M., Moore, J., Lorig, K. *et al.* (1998) A randomized trial of a lay-led self-management group intervention for back pain patients in primary care. *Spine* **23**(23): 2608–2615.

Wagner, E.H., Austin, B.T., Davis, C., Hindmarsh, M., Schaefer, J., Bonomi, A.E. (2001) Improving chronic illness care: translating evidence into action. *Health Affairs* **20**(6): 64–78.

Wagner, E., Austin, B., Von Korff, M. (1996) Organizing care for patients with chronic illness. *The Milbank Quarterly* **74**(4): 511–542.

Walker, C., Peterson, C.L., Millen, N., Martin, C. (2003) *Chronic Illness: New Perspectives and New Directions*. Tertiary Press: Croydon.

Wanless, D. (2002) *Securing our Future Health: Taking a Long Term View*. HM Treasury: London.

Warsi, A., Wang, P.S., LaValley, M.P., Avorn, J., Solomon, D.H. (2004) Self-management education programs in chronic disease. *Archives of Internal Medicine* **164**(9/23): 1641–1649.

Weiss, R. (1973) *Loneliness: The Experience of Emotional and Social Isolation*. MIT Press: Cambridge, MA.

Whitby, B. (2003) A framework for a systematic approach to chronic condition self-management in South Australia. *Guiding Us Forward: National Chronic Condition Self-management Conference*. Australian Government Department of Health & Ageing: Melbourne.

Wilcocks, A. (2001) *Occupation for Health: A Journey from Self Health to Prescription*. British College of Occupational Therapists/Lavenham Press: London.

Wilkinson, R., Marmot, M. (2003) *Social Determinants of Health: The Solid Facts*, 2nd edition. World Health Organization: Europe.

Wilson, P.M. (2001) A policy analysis of the expert patient in the United Kingdom: self-care as an expression of pastoral power? *Health and Social Care in the Community* **9**(3): 134–142.

World Health Organization. (1986) Ottawa Charter for Health Promotion. *International Conference on Health Promotion and Canadian Public Health Association*, Ottawa.

World Health Organization. (2002) *Innovative Care for Chronic Conditions: Building Blocks for Action: Global Report*. World Health Organization: Geneva.

6. *The Relevance of Self-Management Programmes for People with Chronic Disease at Risk for Disease-Related Complications*

Barbara Paterson and Max Hopwood

Introduction

In the past 20 years, there has been a surge of interest among health-care funders, practitioners and researchers in regard to the prevention of disease-related complications in chronic illness (Knight *et al.* 2006). Such complications are widely acknowledged to cause considerable disruption to people with chronic diseases and excessive demands on the health-care system. The focus of most preventive efforts in this regard has been to teach, support and motivate people to become effective self-managers of their disease by their participation in self-management interventions.

Despite a plethora of self-management interventions in recent years, research, particularly in the United States and the United Kingdom, has documented low recruitment yields, high rates of attrition and a relatively low level of participation in self-management interventions (Griffiths *et al.* 2005; Gucciardi *et al.* 2007). There is general acknowledgement that some people are harder to attract to self-management interventions than others, particularly people of low socio-economic status and marginalised populations (Gross 2006). Researchers have demonstrated that those most likely to attend self-management interventions are well-resourced in terms of finances, education and support (Thoolen *et al.* 2007a). The participation of only highly select populations in self-management interventions has resulted in a field of knowledge that does not represent those most at risk for disease-related complications, such as the poor, the elderly and marginalised populations (Chodosh *et al.* 2005; Decoster & Cummings 2005; Taylor & Bury 2007). Gross and Fogg (2001) remind us that when the requirements outweigh the perceived benefits of the intervention, people who are enrolled in an intervention are likely to drop out or not to participate in the intervention. Many questions remain about the appeal and relevance of such interventions in the real-world of people with chronic illnesses who are at risk for disease-related complications.

This chapter is a synthesis of published international research about self-management interventions within the field of type 2 diabetes. Unlike meta-analyses and systematic reviews that have been previously conducted (e.g. Norris *et al.* 2002; Weingarten *et al.* 2002; Jack 2003; Ismail *et al.* 2004; Wantland *et al.* 2004; Leeman 2006), we do not intend to generate conclusions about the effectiveness of specific interventions or to critique the research design. Instead, we wish to provide an overview of the self-management education and/or behavioural support interventions that have been reported in the published literature for the purpose of revealing how the way the interventions have been framed by researchers has influenced who chooses to participate and to remain in the intervention. We have opted to focus on subject participation as evidenced by the profile of the samples in self-management intervention research, including those who leave the intervention or those who do not participate fully in it.

In this chapter, we will propose that the failure of many self-management interventions to address the needs of those most at risk for disease-related complications accounts, in part, for the fairly homogenous population that has been attracted to the interventions, as well as for the attrition to be high. Further, we will suggest that the participation of high-risk populations may be enhanced if such programmes are developed and implemented according to the principles of harm reduction. We will conclude with a discussion of the implications of this synthesis for future research and clinical practice in the field of chronic illnesses.

Background

Despite numerous meta-analyses and systematic reviews about the evaluation of self-management interventions, it is not clear as to what elements of these interventions guarantee success in achieving effective self-management. Weingarten and colleagues (2002) determined that over a hundred different interventions, both lay and practitioner led, achieved similar outcomes. This suggests that it is the decision to participate in a self-management intervention, not the mode of the intervention, which is the key to its effectiveness (Taylor & Bury 2007). However, a number of features of self-management interventions have been identified as resulting in the most consistently positive outcomes. These include tailoring of the intervention to the cultural group and providing community educators or lay people as leaders, as well as individualised assessment, behavioural support, feedback and more than 10 contact times delivered over more than 26 months. Interventions that are commonly associated with poorer outcomes include those that use mainly didactic teaching or those that focus only on disease knowledge (Glazier *et al.* 2006).

In general, self-management interventions share many of the same challenges regarding recruitment and retention that are common in randomised controlled trials (RCTs) of educational and behavioural support interventions. There is an under-representation of younger (under 35) and elderly (over 65) adults, ethnic minorities and people with low levels of education (Thoolen *et al.* 2007a). There is also a tendency to recruit people who are well educated and have the desire and ability to attend a series of intensive education classes (Glasgow 1991; Clark & Hampson 2001). Anderson *et al.* (2005) determined that both the control and experimental groups in their evaluation study demonstrated small to modest improvements in outcomes in a diabetes self-management intervention. They indicated that this was largely because the intervention was attractive to those who had a previous commitment to self-management.

Several reviews have focused on the characteristics of those who selected not to participate in intervention research trials (Hunninghake *et al.* 1987; Glasgow *et al.* 1991; Torgerson *et al.* 1996; Featherstone & Donovan 1998; Ross *et al.* 1999; Ellis 2000; Froehlicher & Lorig 2002; Toobert *et al.* 2003). The most commonly cited reasons for refusal to participate in such RCTs are lack of time, lack of interest or motivation and uncertainty about the effectiveness and requirements of the intervention (Thoolen *et al.* 2007a). In an analysis of attrition in one self-management intervention study, researchers (Thoolen *et al.* 2007a) discovered that most frequently participants left the intervention due to practical reasons, such as lack of transportation. Participants in some self-management intervention studies have cited family or work demands, lack of transportation and time conflicts as being the barriers contributing to the attrition in self-management interventions (Noel *et al.* 1998; Banister *et al.* 2004; Rosal *et al.* 2005). Those who are employed full- or part-time are more likely, than the unemployed, to refuse to participate in self-management interventions, perhaps because most interventions are offered during day hours in the regular work week (Gucciardi *et al.* 2007).

There is conflicting evidence about the influence of language and cultural heritage on participation and retention rates in self-management interventions. People who do not speak English have been shown in some studies to be less likely to participate in self-management interventions in predominantly English-speaking countries (Carter *et al.* 1996; Karter *et al.* 2000; Bruce *et al.* 2003). However, other research has indicated that participation and retention rates are high in self-management interventions delivered in a culturally relevant and language-specific manner (Anderson *et al.* 1991; Balamurugan *et al.* 2006; Gucciardi *et al.* 2007). Literacy is another factor that influences participation and attrition in self-management interventions. Interventions that require reading and/or writing are unlikely to attract and retain people with low levels of literacy (Balamurugan *et al.* 2006), particularly in interventions requiring reading, writing, reflection or group discussions (Torgerson *et al.* 1996; Ellis 2000; Thoolen *et al.* 2007a).

There is limited evidence that suggests that a person's participation in self-management intervention research is influenced by the treatment for the disease and the time since diagnosis. In one type 2 diabetes self-management intervention study, Thoolen *et al.* (2007a) determined that participation rates varied according to the intensity of the person's diabetes treatment and the time since diagnosis. People receiving intensive treatment were more likely to be attracted to and remain in an intervention early on in their disease, and people receiving the usual care were more likely to participate some years after the diagnosis.

Authors have questioned whether self-management is a goal for some people with chronic illness, particularly those with low health literacy and those who wish to assume a passive role in which they do as their health-care provider tells them (Gazmararian *et al.* 2003). Recently, there have been concerted efforts to address the limitations of self-management interventions in reaching populations most at risk for disease-related complications, particularly those who live in poverty and those who are members of an at-risk minority group (e.g. African Americans). Interventions specifically targeted to these at-risk groups have included culturally relevant teaching strategies and involved members of the targeted community as peer educators and/or supports.

Theoretical framework

Preventing disease-related complications is preventing the harm associated with risk behaviours in living with a chronic disease, such as ignoring the dietary guidelines of disease management. The theoretical framework for this chapter is the harm reduction theory in accordance with the modern harm reduction movement, an approach to health risk management that is historically linked to the field of illicit drugs. Harm reduction principles are typically held as synonymous with the reduction of drug-related harm. We believe, however, that it may be possible to apply these principles more widely. As Myers *et al.* (2004) suggest, harm reduction theory may contribute to an enhanced understanding of issues that influence people's engagement in health behaviours, as well as promote the use of community empowerment approaches in disease prevention that extend beyond traditional ones. In this chapter, we refer to 'harm' in chronic illness as the disease-related complications that are known to be linked to risk behaviours.

Lenton and Single (1998) have proposed a socio-political definition of harm reduction. Consistent with this definition are principles used to guide harm reduction interventions for people living with chronic illness (Single 1995; Lenton & Single 1998). The essence of harm reduction, according to this definition, is the recognition that the intervention must start from the client's needs and personal goals, and that all change that reduces the harms associated with risky behaviour is regarded as valuable (Tatarsky 2003). This means that small incremental positive changes towards health goals are seen as steps in the right direction.

Applying this definition to a broader context of chronic illness, we consider any intervention to be consistent with the aims of harm reduction if it (a) has a primary goal of the reduction of harm rather than compliance to the prescribed regime; (b) allows for the inclusion of strategies for those people who continue unhealthy or risky practices; and (c) is likely to produce an overall reduction in harm for an individual. The values and principles of harm reduction are centred on pragmatism wherein the central aim is to control the consequences and reduce the harms of specific behaviours, not to eliminate the behaviours (Tatarsky 2003). Harm reduction applies humanistic values of respect and dignity to therapeutic relationships and, through a collaborative and iterative health professional–patient negotiation, prioritises the needs and diverse perspectives of individuals (Brocato & Wagner 2003; Hayhow & Lowe 2006).

Overview of relevant research

The research question that guided this review was, 'What assumptions and understandings about how people are motivated and prepared to engage in self-management interventions are revealed within the design and implementation of self-management interventions and within the profile of those who enrol, remain or leave the intervention?' Because type 2 diabetes is one of the most common chronic diseases affecting adults in all nations (Clark & Hampson 2001) and diabetes-related complications have been a popular focus for many self-management interventions, we decided that the question could be best addressed in a synthesis of published literature about self-management interventions in type 2 diabetes. Self-management of type 2 diabetes is widely acknowledged to be significant in preventing the disease-related complications of ischaemic heart disease, renal disease and visual impairment (Chodosh *et al.* 2005). It is estimated that only a quarter of those referred to self-management interventions for type 2 diabetes attend, and of those who do attend as many as 57% leave the intervention prematurely (Gucciardi *et al.* 2007).

Sample

The criteria for selection of the body of research (i.e. primary research studies) included in this synthesis were research reports, published in refereed journals and written in English within the past decade (1998–2008), in which (a) the intervention was designed to foster effective self-management of type 2 diabetes among adults; (b) one of the measured outcomes was glycosylated haemoglobin (HbA1c); and (c) there was data about participation and/or attrition in the sample. We included all the studies that met our inclusion criteria and not just the randomised controlled trials because quasi-experimental and comparative studies might reveal salient insights (Mühlhauser & Berger 2002). We did not select literature that referred to interventions focused on single self-management tasks (e.g. foot care) or those that targeted both type 1 and type 2 diabetes. We also excluded research that included large-scale diabetes clinical intervention trials, such as the Diabetes Control and Complications Trial (DCCT) in the United States. While many of these have been successful in achieving significant improvements in glycemic control, they involve large and highly selective populations, costly services involving multidisciplinary approaches and long-term involvement from both the participants and practitioners (Stetson *et al.* 2006).

Thirty-four primary research studies met our criteria for inclusion; they assessed the outcomes of 42 interventions. The description of the interventions, as well as the sample profile and rates of participation and attrition are represented in Table 6.1. Twenty-three of the research studies were RCTs; the remainder had quasi-experimental designs. The majority of the research originated from the United States ($n = 22$); the remainder emanated from the United Kingdom ($n = 3$), Sweden ($n = 3$), Japan ($n = 1$), Canada ($n = 1$), Germany ($n = 1$), the Netherlands ($n = 1$) and Korea ($n = 2$). The research was conducted within the health profession disciplines, primarily medicine and nursing.

There are a number of noteworthy attributes about this body of research. In all but a few studies, the intervention was designed by practitioners/researchers and it is not apparent that people with diabetes have been consulted in the development of the intervention. Most studies have been conducted by teams of researchers within urban academic centres or tertiary hospitals. The interventions they describe are generally resource-intensive and require considerable time commitment from the participants and/or interventionists. There is limited research that reflects the experience of people with type 2 diabetes who live in rural and remote regions, are not well-educated, live in poverty and represent particular minority populations (e.g. Aboriginals).

Sample profile

With the exception of the 13 studies that targeted particular minority groups, the sample population in the primary research studies was remarkably homogenous. Most participants were women over 55 years of age, partnered, with education at high school level or above and diagnosed with diabetes of more than 6 years. The majority of studies that were conducted in the United States included participants who had medical insurance; being insured was an inclusion criterion for 13 of these 23 studies. Some researchers (Raji *et al.* 2002; Steed *et al.* 2005; Young *et al.* 2005; Cho *et al.* 2006; Kulzer *et al.* 2007) reported that the majority of participants in their research were men, although the difference in numbers of women and men in the sample was often slight (1–5%). The predominance of males in this body of research may be explained, in part, by the recruitment strategies in these studies. Raji *et al.* (2002), for example, recruited their participants from a predominantly male Veterans Hospital.

A significant element of the sample profile in this body of research is the baseline HbA1c levels of the participants, reported in all but four of the primary research reports. The baseline HbA1c level is the most significant factor influencing the effect size of self-management interventions designed to improve glycaemic control and prevent disease-related complications (Sigurdardottir *et al.* 2007). Seventeen of the 31 studies indicated that the sample had baseline HbA1c levels within or slightly above the target range ($n = 13$ with baseline HbA1c below 7.4; $n = 4$ with baseline HbA1c below 8.0). Four of the five studies that reported mean baseline HbA1c levels above 9.0 were conducted with Mexican or African Americans. Raji *et al.* (2002) proposed that the high numbers of people in their sample who had HbA1c levels within the target range would suggest that these people had already made a commitment to self-management and thus were prepared to engage in a self-management intervention.

In many studies, the participants were to some degree a 'captive audience'. For example, in the study by Levetan *et al.* (2002), participants were completing an American Diabetes Association (ADA)-recognised diabetes education programme. Because such people have already demonstrated their commitment to self-management by enrolment in the diabetes education programme, they may have been unlikely to decline participation in a further intervention that promised to enhance what they were learning.

The interventions

The interventions represented in the primary research ranged from 3 to 52 hours in duration (mean = 15.3 hours). They were conducted mainly in urban classrooms in settings such as clinics or hospitals ($n = 25$). Some ($n = 7$) were offered in community settings. For example, Brown *et al.* (2002, 2005, 2007) provided sessions to Mexican Americans with type 2 diabetes in settings such as churches, schools, participants' homes or adult day centres. Most interventions were structured to be provided on a schedule determined solely by the researchers. A few researchers (Brown *et al.* 2002, 2005, 2007; Tang *et al.* 2005) offered flexibility to participants by providing multiple sessions for participants to access.

Five interventions involved an online or computer-generated intervention and five others used the telephone to deliver advice/support to people with diabetes. All but six of the 42 interventions entailed a structured curriculum, script or protocol, developed by a team of researchers and/or health-care practitioners. The exceptions to this (Glasgow *et al.* 2002, 2003, 2006; Keyserling *et al.* 2002; Gary *et al.* 2003; Tang *et al.* 2005) delivered content in the intervention that was determined primarily by the nature of the concerns and interests of the participants. These interventions did not always focus entirely on self-management. Gary *et al.* (2003), for example, indicated that in 77% of the intervention visits health-care practitioners addressed other issues such as finances, family responsibilities, insurance and other concerns.

The 42 interventions were primarily educational in their focus, although two (Williams *et al.* 2005; Bradshaw *et al.* 2007) were designed to provide only behavioural support in self-management. Teaching in the educational interventions was primarily delivered in group or individual sessions by a health-care practitioner. For example, Skelly *et al.* (2005) employed nurses to provide an in-home symptom-focused self-management teaching intervention consisting of four modules to participants in their homes. Six studies (Brown *et al.* 2002, 2005, 2007; Keyserling *et al.* 2002; Gary *et al.* 2003; Two Feathers *et al.* 2005) used community members as peer supports and/or educators in the intervention. Three (Brown *et al.* 2002; Skinner *et al.* 2006; Gucciardi *et al.* 2007) invited family members to attend.

Twenty of the educational interventions used only didactic teaching methods. Others added peer support, goal-setting, practice exercises and/or telephone or in-person feedback. Adolfsson *et al.* (2007), for example, included short- and long-term goal setting exercises within their classroom education sessions. The details of goal-setting approaches were largely absent in the primary research that indicated that goal-setting had been an element of the intervention. Researchers typically used phrases such as 'reciprocal goal-setting' to describe goal setting but did not explicate what this entailed.

Some interventions ($n = 12$) were specifically designed to attract and meet the needs of minority groups who were at high risk for diabetes complications (i.e. African Americans, Hispanic Americans, Mexican Americans, Portugese Canadians, Chinese Americans). Although these interventions were described by the researchers as 'culturally tailored' to the target population, only Brown *et al.* (2002, 2005, 2007), Anderson-Loftin *et al.* (2005) and Keyserling *et al.* (2000, 2002) described how they consulted members of the target group by conducting interviews to determine what they would deem as culturally relevant interventions and research processes.

Participation

Nine primary research reports included a discussion of how participants assigned to the intervention group attended the intervention. For example, Adolfsson *et al.* (2007) noted that only 69% of the 50 participants in the intervention group attended each of the five educational sessions. Likewise, Tang *et al.* (2005) report that approximately half of the participants in their study attended less than two-thirds of the scheduled sessions in the intervention. Cho *et al.* (2006) tracked participation in their online intervention by noting the number of times participants logged onto the system. Half of the participants logged onto the system less than twice a week, and 20% averaged no more than two to three times a month.

A few researchers (Brown *et al.* 2005; Mauldon *et al.* 2006) asked participants for feedback about why they did not attend all intervention sessions. The main reasons for lack of attendance were being too busy, conflicts with work schedules, needing transportation, travel/moving or child care issues. Mauldon *et al.* (2006) found that some participants were unable to attend morning classes because of competing work schedules and were required to use their vacation time from work to attend the intervention. However, Tang *et al.* (2005) discovered that morning sessions attracted more participants (mean of 16 participants) than those offered in the afternoon (mean = 8). The relationship between participation and attrition rate was not explored in any of the research reports.

Attrition

Attrition statistics were reported in all of the primary research reports; however, most researchers reported overall attrition in the study and did not refer specifically to attrition within the intervention group. The rates of attrition varied from 1 to 39.2% but it was not always clear how the researchers calculated these figures. For example, Cho *et al.* (2006) report that the attrition in the intervention group was 11% but did not include the five participants who were withdrawn from the study because of inadequate data (e.g. they did not visit the diabetes centre more than three times over 2 years) in that calculation.

Attrition was highest in interventions that were solely educational and required considerable time commitments from the participants (e.g. Sarkadi & Rosen-qvist 2004; Skinner *et al*. 2006). It was lowest in interventions in which the content/process of the intervention had been determined on the basis of feed-back from the target population and the teachers included community peers (e.g. Brown *et al*. 2002, 2005, 2007), or where the content was determined by the needs and interests of participants (e.g. Glasgow *et al*. 2003; Mauldon *et al*. 2006).

Four primary research studies (Williams *et al*. 2005; Skinner *et al*. 2006; Kulzer *et al*. 2007; Thoolen *et al*. 2007b) conducted post hoc analyses to determine whether particular demographic or research variables were associated with attrition. Kulzer *et al*. (2007) reported no differences in the characteristics of those who withdrew from the intervention and those who remained. Skinner *et al*. (2006) and Williams *et al*. (2005) determined that the participants who left the intervention were younger than those who stayed. Williams *et al*. (2005) found that those who left were less likely to be married or partnered, had diabetes for a shorter time and had higher baseline HbA1c levels than their counterparts who remained. Thoolen *et al*. (2007b) determined that the participants who left the intervention were less educated than those who completed the intervention. While the attempt to differentiate between those who left the intervention and those who remained is laudable, it is important to acknowledge that the intervention may be viewed differently by those who choose to participate and those who do not (Hunninghake *et al*. 1987). None of the researchers report asking the participants who left for their views on the intervention.

Researchers in eight studies asked participants to indicate why they left the intervention. Wang and Chan (2005) report that because the classes were held dur-ing a traditional Chinese holiday season, 7 of the 40 Chinese American participants left because of holiday travel plans. The most common responses to questions about the reason for attrition were work or child care conflicts, travel, discontent with content or process of intervention, illness/surgery, moving/migrating and personal obligations or problems. Many of these reasons are consistent with what we know about the complex and crisis-oriented lives of people with diabetes who lack resources, education and supports and are most at risk for diabetes-related complications (Gross *et al*. 2001).

A few researchers (Steed *et al*. 2005; Anderson-Loftin *et al*. 2005; Adolfsson *et al*. 2007; Thoolen *et al*. 2007b) noted when attrition had occurred in the intervention. Interestingly, Adolfsson *et al*. (2007) and Steed *et al*. (2005) indicate that some participants withdrew immediately prior to the intervention, despite having given consent to participate in the study. Thoolen *et al*. (2007b) stipulate that 20 participants who had provided informed consent were unable to participate in the intervention because of transportation difficulties. Attrition also occurred after the initial sessions of the intervention in studies by Adolfsson *et al*. (2007), Thoolen *et al*. (2007b), Anderson-Loftin *et al*. (2005) and Steed *et al*. (2005). This suggests that there may have been aspects of the intervention, such as requiring the person to come to an urban centre during work hours, which were significant in the participant's decision to withdraw.

A limitation of the synthesis provided in this chapter is that it is difficult, if not impossible, to decipher if those who left the intervention, or did not participate fully in it, did so because of an aversion to research or because they found the intervention unsatisfactory or irrelevant. There is a considerable body of research that indicates that people of racial/ethnic minorities tend to hold negative attitudes towards participating in research, particularly in relation to prevention interventions (Giuliano *et al.* 2000; Kressin *et al.* 2000; Shavers *et al.* 2002). However, most primary researchers who asked participants for their reasons for attrition related the same to personal and intervention factors, not participation in the research.

Discussion

In this chapter, we have presented a synthesis of published research about self-management interventions in type 2 diabetes as a means of illustrating that people who are most at risk for disease-related complications are unlikely to be attracted to or to remain in such intervention programmes. The synthesis of primary research has presented a general profile of people with type 2 diabetes attracted to self-management interventions as middle-aged Caucasian people who are highly motivated and interested in improving their self-management, as well as well-resourced in terms of support, finances and education. Even within this sample population the attrition rates are higher and the participation rates lower than is ideal. What is most disturbing about this profile, however, is the question of who is not represented, that is, who is not attracted to and retained in the intervention. One must conclude that self-management interventions are missing a significant proportion of people who are at risk for diabetes-related complication. This is an undesirable situation that needs to be addressed. The tenets of harm reduction theory can shed light on how interventionists can effectively address this phenomenon.

Ensuring the voice of people with chronic illness

The active engagement of illicit drug users (IDUs) in the design, implementation and evaluation of prevention interventions has become an important feature of harm reduction initiatives involving IDUs (Moskalewicz *et al.* 2007). Such engagement is viewed as an expression of horizontal relationships and partnership between practitioners and IDUs where IDUs are active partners and not passive recipients (Moskalewicz *et al.* 2007). There has been a recent onslaught of self-management interventions that seek to involve the person with chronic illness as an active participant in setting goals and determining ways to solve problems in self-management (Jack 2003). Such a step is increasingly acknowledged to be necessary to ensure participation of those most at risk for disease-related complications (Griffin *et al.* 2000).

Despite the fact that some interventions included opportunities for the participant to engage in individual goal setting exercises and others included people with diabetes as peer educators, the voice of the person with chronic disease is remarkably absent in the primary research synthesised in this chapter. In keeping with the findings of other reviews (Jack *et al.* 2004; Newbould *et al.* 2006), the majority of interventions in the primary research were led by health-care practitioners. Even those that purported to involve people with chronic illness in mutual goal-setting and/or as peer mentors were developed exclusively by practitioners. The topics to be reviewed, the approaches to be used and the peer educators were selected by the practitioners with limited or no input from people with chronic illness.

The determination of the intervention by health-care practitioners is problematic at many levels. It presupposes that the health-care practitioner knows best what is good and right for the person with chronic illness. Considerable evidence exists that people who live with a chronic illness develop self-management approaches that work for them; these are often not located in any health professional textbook (Paterson *et al.* 2001). The self-management interventions that are designed solely by health-care practitioners run the risk of actually interfering with the authoritative knowledge that the ill person has developed over time about what works best for him or her and under what circumstances. Such an approach may also convey paternalism and a discounting of the ill person's authoritative knowledge.

Models exist of how people with chronic disease could be more involved as partners in decisions about the design, implementation and evaluation of self-management interventions. Brown *et al.* (2002, 2005, 2007) have included videotapes of Mexican Americans in real-life community settings in educational sessions. They also conducted research with Mexican Americans to determine their preferences for the structure and process of the intervention before the intervention was designed. Although such research has been beneficial in providing foundational support for the relevance of interventions to people with chronic illness, it has not been particularly illuminating in determining what motivates people to participate in self-management interventions. We know little about why some people within a specific population do not participate in culturally tailored interventions.

Most of the primary research represented within this chapter has engaged people with chronic disease primarily as research subjects, and not as partners. Consequently, the success of the interventions has been determined largely on the basis of indicators of changed behaviour or attitudes that interventionists believe are markers of intervention success. What participants think about the intervention, including its relevance and accessibility, is overlooked for the most part.

The voice of those who have chosen not to participate or to leave the intervention is silent in this body of research. Post hoc analyses by demographic categories have not greatly enhanced our understanding about why individuals from certain groups choose to terminate participation in a self-management intervention. Variables, such as the educational level, provide little meaningful insights about those who dropped out and their experience with the intervention (Gross *et al.* 2001). For example, post hoc analyses do not answer why people who are younger, unpartnered and with lower levels of education drop out at higher rates than others. Is it that lack of partner support, less education and a younger age that makes one less motivated? Are these people more likely to be employed in jobs with little autonomy and flexibility, limiting their ability to attend intervention programmes? Might the goals for participating in self-management intervention programmes be different among those who do not have a partner, have less education and younger than among those who are partnered, older and well-educated?

It is possible that the reason for people with particular demographic characteristics to leave the intervention is found not in the personal characteristics but within the intervention's structure or processes (Motzer *et al.* 1997). Participants may drop out of self-management interventions because the incentives for participation are not sufficient enough or of the right kind to entice them to remain, particularly when the person is also faced with a myriad of competing responsibilities such as those related to work, school and children (Gross *et al.* 2001). In addition, it is possible that participants stop coming to self-management intervention programmes because the programme goals do not complement their personal goals.

Gross *et al.* (2001) describe a model of engagement of parents in parenting interventions in which they asked parents to identify their motivations for participation and their responses to a variety of incentives after they had provided informed consent to participate in the research. They make the point that we need to find out from people who have agreed to participate how they made such a decision and what incentives were meaningful to them. They emphasise that by building a body of research about which interventional structures, processes and content work and with whom, we can expect that interventionists will make better decisions about how to construct intervention programmes that people want to attend.

Compassionate pragmatism

The philosophical underpinnings of harm reduction lie in *compassionate pragmatism* whereby harm reductionists meet people 'where they are' in terms of their life situations, readiness, needs and personal goals (Marlatt & Kilmer 1998). There is an acknowledgement that the one-size-fits-all approach does not work because people are so varied in their needs, goals, supports, resources, past experiences and values (Tatarsky 2003). The compassionate pragmatist also recognises that not all people are willing or able to cease their risk practices. This translates into the need for accepting goals for harm reduction other than the avoidance of risk behaviours, while at the same time striving towards risk avoidance. It also requires harm reduction approaches that are flexible enough to meet the needs of the circumstances and goals of individual participants (Tatarsky 2003).

Understanding why many people at risk for disease-related complications do not participate is critical to addressing the issue of low participation rates in self-management interventions. Firstly, both recruitment and retention of people with chronic illness in self-management interventions are influenced by the perspective they hold about living with the disease. Perspectives about living with chronic illness encapsulates the beliefs, expectations and values that people hold about living with the disease (Paterson 2001). People who live with chronic illness and attempt to maintain a wellness in the foreground perspective may strive to put the disease and its sequelae in the background of their lives in order that they can live as normally as possible (Paterson 2001; Taylor & Bury 2007). They may resist any programme that requires them to focus on the negative aspects of living with the disease, such as the possibility of disease-related complications. The intervention itself may precipitate a shift to the illness in the foreground perspective, causing participants to leave the programme in response.

There are numerous personal, social, economic, cultural and political factors that constrain people's ability to engage in self-management. Liebman *et al.* (2007), for example, concluded that the most significant factor affecting participation in a programme of self-management activities was the lack of space and other resources for the programme, not the commitment of the participants to self-management. For some, an intervention that is framed to assist the person to comply with a prescribed regime is seen as requiring submission to authority. Because of past clashes with people in authority or personal makeup, such an intervention may be viewed as something to be avoided (Paterson *et al.* 2001; Tatarsky 2003). For others, risk practices may hold personal meaning and may be considered beneficial (e.g. eating high carbohydrate foods as an integral part of cultural holidays). Any intervention that promises to alter such risk practices may be met with anxiety and resistance.

Another factor that determines the person's willingness to participate in self-management interventions is the nature and quality of the person's relationship with the health-care practitioner or peer who is providing the intervention (Gotler *et al.* 2000). However, no research that included interventions delivered by health-care practitioners examined this factor in any depth, other than global measures of participant satisfaction with the intervention. The significance of this omission was illustrated in a study by Uitewaal *et al.* (2004) in which the researchers assessed outcomes of a diabetes programme that was tailored to Turkish people in the Netherlands and provided by Turkish educators. They determined that 36% of the participants (31% of the men, 39% of the women) did not particularly identify themselves with the educator. This further influenced the participants' assessment of the effectiveness and relevance of the intervention.

A supportive collaborative approach is often an effective way to develop a person's motivation to learn more about diabetes self-management, possibly in a formalised self-management intervention programme. Such a moderated approach avoids the 'comply or rebel' bind (Tatarsky 2003) that interventions with a singular view of what is good and right in self-management perpetuate. This does not mean that people with chronic illness cannot entertain goals of ideal self-management or that they are not capable of achieving such a goal. Rather, by accepting a person's goals for living with a disease as a legitimate starting point, practitioners provide an opportunity for people with chronic illness to engage with a practitioner in an alliance that may lead to the development of further goals.

Countering healthism

On the heel of globalisation emerged a new consumer movement and health consciousness that sociologist Robert Crawford (1980) refers to as 'healthism'. Consistent with the neo-liberal focus on individualism, healthism construes individual behaviour, attitudes and emotions as the factors that need attention for the realisation of health, and solutions to preventing or managing illness are seen to lie in the realm of individual choice. For proponents of this new health consciousness the path to good health is via self-regulation – an individual's determination to resist the temptations of culture and advertising, to overcome institutional and environmental constraints, to resist disease agents and to refuse to accept lazy or poor personal habits. Individuals are implored to take personal responsibility by engaging in a variety of practices like exercise, attending to diet and eliminating other risk behaviours (Crawford 1980).

But personal responsibility risks the myopia of classical individualism whereby personal responsibility is seen to be all that anyone ever needs (Crawford 1980). Healthism denies the social and cultural constraints that people with chronic illness experience against 'choosing' healthy practices and life styles. Under a regime of healthism, individuals experience intense social pressures to act in such a way as to minimise the likelihood that their behaviours, motivations and emotions will result in costly ill health; failing to act preventively becomes a sign of social, not just individual, irresponsibility. Under this paradigm, all behaviours, attitudes and emotions that are deemed to put individuals at risk of disease are medicalised and people become morally obliged to correct unhealthy habits. The up-shot of the inter-relationship between economic and cultural changes brought about by globalisation and healthism over past decades is that blame is attached to the shame that defines health-related stigma. Individuals or groups ranging from people with type 2 diabetes to people who use illicit drugs are blamed for their ill health, are construed to constitute a personal or community health risk and are viewed as a drain on resources (Jones *et al.* 1984). Crawford (1980) argues that the ideology of healthism fosters a de-politicisation and therefore undermines the *social* effort to improve health and well-being.

While healthism serves as a benefit for many people who adopt a health-promoting life style, it can reinforce an illusion that we, as individuals, always control our own existence and that 'personal action to improve health will somehow satisfy the longing for a much more varied complex of needs' (Crawford 1980, p. 368). Unlike healthism, harm reduction principles acknowledge that not everyone is effective at self-regulating or is in an economic and social position to always prioritise personal health above other considerations. Harm reduction is a philosophy largely born of the experience of social and economic marginalisation and a significant strength of the paradigm is that it acknowledges a wide diversity of people, their beliefs and values within its framework. There are strong parallels between drug dependence and chronic illness, in the sense that people in either circumstance are dealing with entrenched habits that can be damaging to the health and difficult to change (Hayhow & Lowe 2006). Harm reduction policies, programmes and interventions can be tailored to the needs and diverse perspectives of people living with chronic illnesses.

The primary focus of self-management interventions in type 2 diabetes has been on knowledge and skill acquisition. Most of the interventions reviewed in this chapter are based on the assumption that if people know about the disease and its management, they will develop the self-efficacy they need to manage the disease effectively. Self-efficacy has been criticised as reflecting a capitalist 'American dream' (Taylor & Bury 2007) mentality about individual goal achievement that has little relevance in other cultural contexts. There is a lack of empirical evidence to support the notion that self-efficacy is the key to self-management of chronic disease. In addition, the most significant hazard of the focus on self-efficacy is that it perpetuates a narrow view of self-management – one that places the onus for perseverance and other socially accepted norms of successful self-management squarely on the shoulders of people with chronic illness (Taylor & Bury 2007). The influence of social determinants of health and other factors (e.g. paternalistic practitioners who negate the ability of the patient to self-manage the disease) can then be discounted by practitioners and policymakers alike.

Hayhow and Lowe's (2006) discussion of health professionals' objections to harm reduction in chronic disease management highlight conventional views within medicine regarding the importance of adhering to best practice in chronic illness. Magnusson (2004) and Roe (2005) observe that harm reductionists include a variety of middle-class educated health professionals like specialist physicians, academics and policymakers, many of whom are comfortable working within existing institutions, policy and laws 'even though the health problems they address are substantially created by the ideology of systems in which they work' (Roe 2005, p. 245). Similar tensions may arise where harm reduction principles are deployed in chronic disease management. However, the integration of harm reduction approaches in chronic illness is not an argument for disbanding best practice with people who are amenable to making lifestyle changes. Rather, harm reduction acknowledges the divergent values of patients around health and that people have a legitimate human right to actively choose the therapeutic responses that suit their circumstances and lifestyle preferences. For some people with chronic illness, conventional best practice involving lifestyle change is an ideal rather than a reality. Some people continue to make unhealthy lifestyle choices for reasons that are rational to them, even when suffering the consequences of earlier poor choices. Harm reduction proponents attempt to recognise and remove personal judgments about individual behaviour and instead focus on ameliorating the negative consequences of unhealthy practice (Lenton & Single 1998).

Conclusion

In this chapter, we have proposed that there is much to be gained from drawing on harm reduction theory to inform plans to increase the participation and retention of people with chronic illness in self-management interventions. We have proposed that respecting that not all people with chronic illness are able or motivated to engage in self-management, while at the same time acknowledging that they may hold goals for living with the disease that do not include self-management, may be achieved by a grassroots, individualised and flexible approach congruent with harm reduction theory. The focus of the intervention will shift from the person's compliance to a collaborative alliance in which interventionist and participant work together towards shared goals that 'feel right' (Tatarsky 2003) for both parties.

Such an approach is likely to attract a larger and more diverse clientele than is currently the profile of participants in self-management interventions. As an umbrella concept, harm reduction suggests that self-management interventions must be individualised, flexible and responsive enough that interventionists can entertain a variety of goals to meet the diverse needs of a population. Such an approach confirms the fallacy of merely 'teaching' people how to manage their disease on an everyday basis without also providing for the relational spaces that are needed to effectively support the person.

There are a number of implications of the findings of this synthesis for future directions in the field. Interventionists who frame a self-management intervention within the harm reduction theory should make this explicit in their first encounters with people with chronic illness at the time of recruitment. This will require that they make clear that they acknowledge that people with chronic illness have personal and other reasons for maintaining risk practices. Harm reductionists acknowledge that any meaningful behavioural change is likely to be two steps forward and one step back. People who tend to avoid or abandon self-management intervention programmes may be attracted to, or remain, in the programme if such a relapse is anticipated and they are supported to recover from such a lapse. Interventionists who draw on harm reduction theory should be trained in the skills of fostering and enacting collaborative alliances as well as those of harm reduction.

Finally, harm reduction advocates will need to empirically demonstrate to skeptical health professionals that harm reduction interventions are the best practice in some contexts of chronic disease management. Both participants and non-participants should be interviewed or surveyed about their reasons for participating/not participating, particularly in regard to their assessment of the intervention.

The synthesis has highlighted the need for researchers to analyse attrition from the intervention separately from that in the study. The implications for future interventions are likely to be different in both types of attrition (Lauby *et al*. 1996). Also, researchers should determine how participation rates are associated with attrition. Likewise, the synthesis provides support for the critique of RCTs to evaluate self-management interventions. There is a need for research designs in addition to RCTs, or perhaps in the place of RCTs, that effectively address the process issues highlighted in this chapter. The emerging 'realist' approach to evaluation (Pawson *et al*. 2005) that seeks to understand how interventions work and why they fail in particular contexts and settings offers direction for alternative research designs in this regard.

Health professionals have often argued that harm reduction condones and promotes unhealthy lifestyles because it addresses the consequences of unhealthy behaviour, rather than the behaviour. In response, we argue that harm reduction strategies in the context of chronic disease management be implemented on an individual basis such that interventions are not universally applied and become widely misunderstood as a tacit approval of unhealthy behaviours or a promotion of such behaviours. In the management of chronic illness, harm reduction policy programmes and interventions can become valuable contributions to health-care best practice.

Table 6.1 Overview of primary research

Authors	Intervention	Participation in intervention	Attrition	Sample
Adolfsson et al. (2007)	Five 2.5-hour group educational sessions over 7 months facilitated by physicians and diabetes specialist nurses. Included short- and long-term goal setting	69% participated in each session; 31% missed one session	19%	Occurred in Sweden Participants (101) mainly female, over 55 years, unemployed and married Baseline HbA1c in intervention group = 7.4
Anderson-Loftin et al. (2005)	Group education about dietary self-management based on cultural norms of diet as determined in prior research. Four weekly classes in diet, five monthly peer-professional group discussions and weekly telephone follow-up by nurse care-manager		22%	Participants (97) African Americans in rural USA Mainly female, unmarried, unemployed, obese, 55+ years, with less than high school education and having diabetes for 10+ years
Bradshaw et al. (2007)	Resiliency training offered in classroom by health practitioner in 10 modules (15 hours)		30%	Participants (67) in urban USA. Mainly female, married, unemployed with college education

(cont.)

Table 6.1 (cont.)

Authors	Intervention	Participation in intervention	Attrition	Sample
Brown *et al.* (2007)	Culturally competent interventions: 1. 24 hours group education +28 hours support groups 2. 16 hours education; 6 hours support group		4.6%	Participants (216) Mexican Americans in urban/suburban USA Mainly female, obese, 50+ years
Brown *et al.* (2005)	See Brown *et al.* (2007) 1. Eight weeks group education + support group sessions 2. Twelve weekly education sessions and 14 support group discussions	26.3% did not attend most sessions; self-reported reasons were business, too lazy, needed transportation or moving/migrating		Participants (114) Mexican Americans in urban/suburban USA. Mainly female, over 50 years, obese, with less than high school education and having diabetes for 10+ years Baseline HbA1c = 11+
Cho *et al.* (2006)	Online glucose monitoring record that included biweekly feedback and counsel from health-care practitioners + outpatient visits every 3 months to receive education and feedback from physician over 2 years	50% logged into system more than 3 time a week; 30% less than twice a week; 20% two to three times per month	12.5%	Participants (80) in urban Korea. Mainly 50+ years Mean HbA1c 7.7

Clark and Hampson (2001)	Motivational interviewing conducted by psychologist in urban diabetes clinic. Patients received copy of goal setting form and complete self-efficacy scale. Nurse made follow-up telephone call in 1 week to monitor progress. Patients received booklet with content of interview reinforced. Visits to nurse for follow-up at 12, 24 and 52 weeks		Participants (166) in urban USA. Mainly 55+ years old, and overweight Baseline HbA1c = 8.42
Gallegos *et al.* (2006)	Six group educational sessions (90 minutes each) and 20 individualised counselling sessions provided by nurse over 50 weeks. Educational sessions took place in nursing school; counselling occurred in participants' homes or by telephone	26.7%	Participants (45) Mexican adults in urban USA

(*cont.*)

Table 6.1 *(cont.)*

Authors	Intervention	Participation in intervention	Attrition	Sample
Gary *et al.* (2003)	Face-to-face 45-minute visits or telephone contacts with a nurse and/or 45 to 60-minute home visits by a community health worker. Visits approximately three times a year with additional contacts as required. Occurred over 2 years		16%	Participants (186) African Americans living in inner city community in USA Mainly female, 55+ years, obese and with a duration of diabetes of 9 years Baseline HbA1c = 8.6
Glasgow *et al.* (2006)	Computer program focusing on aspects of self-management, tailored goal setting and action planning. Health coaches (lay educators) answer questions and help with action plan in two visits. Plan translated into a computer-generated printout for patient and summary sent to physician. At 1 week and 1 month after first visit with coach, the patient receives follow-up telephone call from coach. Tailored health newsletter mailed at 6 weeks		24.8%; 10% by 2 month period	Participants (400) in urban USA Equal numbers of men and women with high levels of education (35% college educated) and income Baseline HbA1c = 7.4

130

Glasgow *et al.* (2003)	Diabetes Network (D-Net) Internet-based self-management project, plus tailored self-management training or peer support components	18% in a year	Participants (*n* = 320) in urban USA Mainly females who had been diagnosed with diabetes for an average of 8 years, had one or more chronic illnesses in addition to diabetes and had either no or extremely limited Internet experience prior to the study
Glasgow *et al.* (2002)	Brief computer-assisted dietary goal setting, followed by self-help components and support by follow-up telephone calls and/or community resources	11%	Participants (*n* = 321) in urban USA Mainly females who were 59+ years, been diagnosed with diabetes for an average of 6.4 years, and had one or more other chronic illnesses
Gucciardi *et al.* (2007)	Individual diabetes education counselling in conjunction with group education (15 hours over 3 consecutive days) provided by Portuguese-speaking health practitioner. Family encouraged to participate. Content and teaching methods culturally congruent	39.3%	Participants (*n* = 87) Portuguese in urban Canada Mainly females, over 55 years, married, unemployed or retired with education over grade 9 and income over \$19,000/year Baseline HbA1c = 7.0

(cont.)

Table 6.1 *(cont.)*

Authors	Intervention	Participation in intervention	Attrition	Sample
Kulzer *et al.* (2007)	A didactic-oriented training programme (treatment A) was compared with a self-management-oriented programme delivered by health practitioner in group sessions (treatment B). The latter programme was compared with a more individualised approach (treatment C)		6.6% Self-reported the following reasons: acute life-threatening illness ($n = 1$); personal problems ($n = 6$); time problems ($n = 2$); left region because of occupational reasons ($n = 1$); no reason given ($n = 2$)	Participants (181) in urban Germany Mainly male, 55+ years, had diabetes for 6.2+ years Baseline HbA1c = 7.8
Mauldon *et al.* (2006)	Culturally appropriate and culturally relevant Spanish-language cognitive-behavioural diabetes self-care educational intervention. Designed for a population with low literacy and educational levels. Consisted of six weekly, 3-hour sessions. Breakfast and lunch provided	94% attended all sessions Schedule of intervention conflicted with work requirements for some	6% Attrition due to difficulties obtaining adequate child care	Participants ($n = 16$) Latino patients in urban USA Mainly females, over 50 years, married, had diabetes for 8+ years, had less than high school education and were employed Baseline HbA1c = 8.9 75% received a one-on-one diabetes education session prior to the intervention

Parchman et al. (2003)	Diabetes education classes in either Spanish or English (2 hours/week for 5 weeks)	29.2%	Participants (n = 428) Hispanic Americans in urban USA Mainly female, over 50 years, with higher than high school education and diagnosed with diabetes for mean of 7.2 years
Piette (2000)	Biweekly automated assessment and self-care assessment telephone calls in Spanish and English with weekly telephone follow-up by diabetes educator (nurse) over 12 months. Participants used calls to report information about their health and self-care and to access self-care education	50% completed 78% of their assessments	11%	Participants (n = 248) primarily English- and Spanish-speaking people in urban USA Mainly female, English-speaking, over 55 years, employed, having income of over $10,00/year, with greater than high school education and diagnosed with diabetes for mean of 7.2 years Baseline HbA1c = 8.8
Sarkadi and Rosenqvist (2004)	12-month group educational programme led by pharmacists, assisted by diabetes nurse educator	15.4% Self-reported reasons: time constraints, deceased, discontent with group and discontent with contents of intervention	Participants (n = 39) in urban Sweden Mainly females who were 65+ years, slightly overweight and had been diagnosed with diabetes for 5.9+ years Baseline HbA1c below target values in more than half of participants

(cont.)

Table 6.1 (*cont.*)

Authors	Intervention	Participation in intervention	Attrition	Sample
Sarkadi and Rosenqvist (2001)	See the practical aspects of diabetes management, such as choice and preparation of food, performing self-monitoring tasks and walks to decrease blood sugar levels were emphasised		26.1% Self-reported reasons: moving away from the town, social obligations and health problems	Participants ($n = 105$) in urban Sweden Mainly females who were 65+ years, married/partnered, slightly overweight and had been diagnosed with diabetes for 6.7+ years Baseline HbA1c below target values in more than half of participants
Shibayama et al. (2007)	Individualised counselling (once a month for 12 months) in a diabetes outpatient clinic conducted by a nurse. Included assessment, goal setting and advice as well as educational materials. Sessions took 8–76 minutes		10%	Participants ($n = 134$) in urban Japan Mainly male who were 50+ years and normal or slightly overweight Baseline mean HbA1c = 7.3
Skelly et al. (2005)	In-home, nurse-delivered, symptom-focused teaching/counselling intervention		12.8%	Participants ($n = 41$) African Americans in rural USA Mainly male, 62+ years with above high school education, living in own home and had medical insurance Baseline HbA1c = 9.1

| Skinner et al. (2006) | The DESMOND programme for individuals newly diagnosed with type 2 diabetes 6 hours of group education, delivered in one of three formats: 1 day, 2 half-days or three 2-hour sessions by educators who were a mixture of registered dieticians, practice nurses or nurse specialists | 35.6% | Participants (*n* = 236) in urban UK + family members

Mainly male, Caucasian, within 6 weeks of diagnosis at onset and 62+ years |
| Williams et al. (2005) | Patient Activation Intervention – RA met for approximately 20 minutes with participants to prompt them to generate and ask questions during each visit to diabetes practitioner 3 times over 12 months. The activation intervention was based on EPIC trials, and was compared to time-matched passive educational viewing of ADA videotapes

Education Intervention – met with RA for 20 minutes prior to three separate appointments over 12 months. Played videotapes | 15%

Participants who did not complete the study (*n* = 35) were younger [48.7 years versus 55.7, $t(225) = 3.42, P < 0.001$], were less likely to be married or living as married (51.4% versus 70.4%, $\chi^2 = 4.88, P < 0.03$), had diabetes for a shorter time [6.3 years versus 10.8 years, $t(221) = 3.18, P < 0.01$], had a higher baseline relative HbA1c | |

(cont.)

Table 6.1 *(cont.)*

Authors	Intervention	Participation in intervention	Attrition	Sample
	from American Association of Diabetes Educators Patient Education Video Series			
Young *et al.* (2005)	PACCTS over 12 months. Patients were called by telecarer (nurse) for approximately 20 minutes a call according to a protocol that determined frequency of calls according to HbA1c level (once every 3 months if HbA1c was <7%; every 7 weeks if it was in range of 7.1–9%; and monthly if it was >9%). Telecarers followed a script that included self-management education, explorations of readiness to change; and reviews of participants' reports about medication use, blood glucose readings and recent HbA1c levels		16% in PACCTS group	Participants (*n* = 332; 195 in control group and 137 in PACCTS group) in urban UK

RA, research assistant; EPIC, expanding patient involvement in care; PACCTS, Proactive call centre treatment support.

References

Adolfsson, E.T., Walker-Engstrom, M.L., Smide, B., Wikblad, K. (2007) Patient education in type 2 diabetes – a randomized controlled 1-year follow-up study. *Diabetes Research and Clinical Practice* 76: 341–350.

Anderson, R.M., Funnell, M.M., Nwankwo, R., Gillard, M.L., Oh, M., Fitzgerald, J.T. (2005) Evaluating a problem-based empowerment program for African Americans with diabetes: results of a randomized controlled trial. *Ethnicity and Disease* 15: 671–678.

Anderson, R.M., Herman, W.H., Davis, J.M., Freedman, R.P., Funnell, M.M., Neighbors, H.W. (1991) Barriers to improving diabetes care for blacks. *Diabetes Care* 14: 605–609.

Anderson-Loftin, W., Barnett, S., Bunn, P., Sullivan, P., Hussey, J., Tavakoli, A. (2005) Soul food light: culturally competent diabetes education. *Diabetes Educator* 31(4): 355–363.

Balamurugan, A., Rivera, M., Jack, L., Allen, K., Morris, S. (2006) Barriers to diabetes self-management education programs in underserved rural Arkansas: implications for program evaluation. *Preventing Chronic Diseases* 3(1). Retrieved 31 December 2007, from http://www.cdc.gov/pcd/issues/2006/jan/05_0129.htm.

Banister, N.A., Jastrow, S.T., Hodges, V., Loop, R., Gillham, M.B. (2004) Diabetes self-management training program in community clinic improves patient outcomes at modest cost. *Journal of the American Dietetic Association* 104: 807–810.

Bradshaw, B.G., Richardson, G.E., Kumpfer, K. *et al.* (2007) Determining the efficacy of a resiliency training approach in adults with type 2 diabetes. *The Diabetes Educator* 33(4): 650–659.

Brocato, J., Wagner, E.F. (2003) Harm reduction: a social work practice model and social justice agenda. *Health and Social Work* 28: 117–125.

Brown, S.A., Blozis, S.A., Kouzekanani, K., Garcia, A.A., Winchell, M., Hanis, C.L. (2005) Dosage effects of diabetes self-management education for Mexican Americans: the Starr County border health initiative. *Diabetes Care* 28(3): 527–532.

Brown, S.A., Blozis, S.A., Kouzekanani, K., Garcia, A.A., Winchell, M., Hanis, C.L. (2007) Health beliefs of Mexican Americans with type 2 diabetes: the Starr County border health initiative. *The Diabetes Educator* 33: 300–308.

Brown, S.A., Garcia, A.A., Kouzekanani, K., Hanis, C.L. (2002) Culturally competent diabetes self-management education for Mexican Americans: the Starr County border health initiative. *Diabetes Care* 25: 259–268.

Bruce, D.G., Davis, W.A., Cull, C.A., Davis, T.M. (2003) Diabetes education and knowledge in patients with type 2 diabetes from the community: the Fremantle Diabetes Study. *Journal of Diabetes Complications* 17(2): 82–89.

Carter, J.S., Pugh, J.A., Monterrosa, A. (1996) Non-insulin dependent diabetes mellitus in minorities in the United States. *Annals of International Medicine* 125(3): 221–232.

Cho, J.-H., Chang, S.-A., Kwon, H.-S. *et al.* (2006) Long-term effect of the internet-based glucose monitoring system on HbA1c reduction and glucose stability: a 30-month follow-up study for diabetes management with a ubiquitous medical care system. *Diabetes Care* 29: 2625–2631.

Chodosh, J., Morton, S.C., Mojica, W. *et al.* (2005) Meta-analysis: chronic disease self-management programs for older adults. *Annals of Internal Medicine* 143: 427–438.

Clark, M., Hampson, S.E. (2001) Implementing a psychological intervention to improve lifestyle self-management in patients with type 2 diabetes. *Patient Education and Counseling* **42**(3): 247–256.

Crawford, R. (1980) Healthism and the medicalization of everyday life. *International Journal of Health Services* **10**: 365–388.

Decoster, V.A., Cummings, S.M. (2005) Helping adults with diabetes. A review of evidence-based intervention evaluations. *Health and Social Work* **30**(3): 259–264.

Ellis, P.M. (2000) Attitudes towards and participation in randomised clinical trials in oncology: a review of the literature. *Annals of Oncology* **11**: 939–945.

Featherstone, K., Donovan, J.L. (1998) Random allocation or allocation at random? Patients' perspectives on participation in a randomised controlled trial. *British Medical Journal* **317**: 1177–1180.

Froehlicher, E.S., Lorig, K. (2002) Editorial: who cares about recruitment anyway? *Patient Education and Counseling* **48**: 97.

Gallegos, E.C., Ovalle-Berúmen, F., Gomez-Meza, M.V. (2006). Metabolic control of adults with type 2 diabetes mellitus through education and counselling. *Journal of Nursing Scholarship* **38**(4): 344–351.

Gary, T.L., Bone, L.R., Hill, M.N. *et al.* (2003) Randomized controlled trial of the effects of nurse case manager and community health worker interventions on risk factors for diabetes-related complications in urban African Americans. *Preventive Medicine* **37**: 23–32.

Gazmararian, J.A., Williams, M.V., Peel, J., Baker, D.W. (2003) Health literacy and knowledge of chronic disease. *Patient Education and Counseling* **51**: 267–275.

Giuliano, A.R., Mokuau, N., Hughes, C. *et al.* (2000) Participation of minorities in cancer research: the influence of structural, cultural, and linguistic factors. *Annals of Epidemiology* **10** (Suppl 8): 22–34.

Glasgow, R.E. (ed.) (1991) *Compliance to Diabetes Regimens: Conceptualization, Complexity, and Determinants.* Raven: New York.

Glasgow, R.E., Boles, S.M., McKay, H.G., Feil, E.G., Barrera, M. (2003) The D-Net diabetes self-management program: long-term implementation, outcomes, and generalization results. *Preventive Medicine* **36**: 410–419.

Glasgow, R.E., Nutting, P.A., Toobert, D.J. *et al.* (2006) Effects of a brief computer-assisted diabetes self-management intervention on dietary, biological and quality-of-life outcomes. *Chronic Illness* **2**(1): 27–38.

Glasgow, R.E., Toobert, D.J., Hampson, S.E. (1991) Participation in outpatient diabetes education program: how many patients take part and how representative are they? *Diabetes Educator* **17**: 376–380.

Glasgow, R.E., Toobert, D.J., Hampson, S.E., Strycker, L.A. (2002) Implementation, generalization and long-term results of the "choosing well" diabetes self-management intervention. *Patient Education and Counseling* **48**: 115–122.

Glazier, R.H., Bajcar, J., Kennie, N.R., Willson, K. (2006) A systematic review of interventions to improve diabetes care in socially disadvantaged populations. *Diabetes Care* **29**(7): 1675–1688.

Gotler, R.S., Flocke, S.A., Goodwin, M.A., Zyzanski, S.J., Murray, T.H., Stange, K.C. (2000) Facilitating participatory decision-making: what happens in real-world community practice? *Medical Care* **38**(12): 1200–1209.

Griffin, J.A., Gilhiland, S.S., Perez, G., Upson, D., Carter, J.S. (2000) Challenges to participating in a lifestyle intervention program: the Native American diabetes project. *The Diabetes Educator* **26**(7): 681–689.

Griffiths, C., Motlib, J., Azad, A. *et al.* (2005) Expert Bangladeshi patients? Randomised controlled trial of a lay-led self-management programme for Bangladeshis with chronic disease. *British Journal of General Practice* **55**(520): 831–837.

Gross, D. (2006) Editorial: a research agenda for understanding participation in clinical research. *Research in Nursing and Health* **29**: 172–175.

Gross, D., Fogg, L. (2001) Clinical trials in the 21st century: the case for participant-centered research. *Research in Nursing and Health* **24**: 530–539.

Gross, D., Julion, W., Fogg, L. (2001) What motivates participation and dropout among low-income urban families of color in a prevention intervention? *Family Relations* **50**(3): 246–254.

Gucciardi, E., DeMelo, M., Lee, R.N., Grace, S.L. (2007) Assessment of two culturally competent diabetes education methods: individual versus individual plus group education in Canadian Portuguese adults with type 2 diabetes. *Ethnicity and Health* **12**(2): 163–187.

Hayhow, B.D., Lowe, M.P. (2006) Addicted to the good life: harm reduction in chronic disease management. *Medical Journal of Australia* **184**: 235–237.

Hunninghake, D.B., Darby, C.A., Probstfield, J.L. (1987) Recruitment experience in clinical trials: literature summary and annotated bibliography. *Controlled Clinical Trials* **8**: 6s–30s.

Ismail, K., Winkley, K., Rabe-Hesketh, S. (2004) Systematic review and meta-analysis of randomized controlled trials of psychological interventions to improve glycaemic control in patients with type 2 diabetes. *The Lancet* **363**: 1589–1597.

Jack, L. (2003) Diabetes self-management education research. *Disease Management and Health Outcomes* **11**(7): 415–428.

Jack, L., Liburd, L., Spencer, T., Airhihenbuwe, C.O. (2004) Understanding the environment in diabetes self-manangement research: an examination of 8 studies in community-based settings. *Annals of Internal Medicine* **149**(11): 964–971.

Jones, E.E., Scott, R.A., Markus, H. (1984) *Social Stigma: The Psychology of Marked Relationships*. W. H. Freeman: New York.

Karter, A.J., Ferrara, A., Darbinian, J.A., Ackerson, L.M., Selby, J.V. (2000) Self-monitoring of blood glucose: language and financial barriers in a managed care population with diabetes. *Diabetes Care* **23**(4): 477–483.

Keyserling, T.C., Ammerman, A.S., Samuel-Hodge, C.D. *et al.* (2000) A diabetes management program for African American women with type 2 diabetes. *Diabetes Educator* **26**: 796–805.

Keyserling, T.C., Samuel-Hodge, C.D., Ammerman, A.S. *et al.* (2002) A randomized trial of an intervention to improve self-care behaviors of African–American women with type 2 diabetes. *Diabetes Care* **25**: 1576–1583.

Knight, K.M., Dornan, T., Bundy, C. (2006) The diabetes educator: trying hard, but must concentrate more on behaviour. *Diabetic Medicine* **23**(5): 485–501.

Kressin, N.R., Meterko, M., Wilson, N.J. (2000) Racial disparities in participation in biomedical research. *Journal of the National Medical Association* **92**(2): 62–69.

Kulzer, B., Hermann, N., Reinecker, S., Haak, T. (2007) Effects of self-management training in type 2 diabetes: a randomized, prospective trial. *Diabetic Medicine* **24**(4): 415–423.

Lauby, J., Kotranski, L., Feighan, K., Collier, K., Semaan, S., Halbert, J. (1996) Effects of intervention attrition and research attrition on the evaluation of an HIV prevention program. *Journal of Drug Issues* **26**(3): 663–667.

Leeman, J. (2006) Interventions to improve diabetes self-management. *The Diabetes Educator* **32**(4): 571–583.

Lenton, S., Single, E. (1998) The definition of harm reduction. *Drug and Alcohol Review* **17**: 213–220.

Levetan, C.S., Dawn, K.R., Robbins, D.C., Ratner, R.E. (2002) Impact of computer-generated personalized goals on HbA1c. *Diabetes Care* **25**: 2–8.

Liebman, J., Heffernan, D., Sarvela, P. (2007) Teaching how, not what: the contributions of community health workers to diabetes self-management. *The Diabetes Educator* **33**(6): 132S–138S.

Magnusson, R.S. (2004) "Underground euthanasia" and the harm minimization debate. *Journal of Law, Medicine and Ethics* **32**: 486–495.

Marlatt, G.A., Kilmer, J.R. (1998). Consumer choice: implications of behavioral economics for drug use and treatment. *Behavior Therapy* **29**(4): 567–576.

Mauldon, M., D'Eramo Melkus, G., Cagganello, M. (2006) A culturally appropriate diabetes education program for Spanish-speaking individuals with type 2 diabetes mellitus – evaluation of a pilot project. *The Diabetes Educator* **32**(5): 751–760.

Moskalewicz, J., Barrett, D., Bujalski, M. *et al.* (2007) Harm reduction coming of age: a summary of the '18th International Conference on the Reduction of Drug Related Harm' – Warsaw, Poland: 13–17 May 2007. *International Journal of Drug Policy* **18**(6): 503–508.

Motzer, S.A., Moseley, J.R., Lewis, F.M. (1997). Recruitment and retention of families in clinical trials with longitudinal designs. *Western Journal of Nursing Research* **19**(3): 314–333

Mühlhauser, I., Berger, M. (2002) Patient education – evaluation of a complex intervention. *Diabetologia* **45**(12): 944–954.

Myers, T., Aggelton, P., Kippax, S. (2004) Perspectives on harm reduction: editorial introduction. *Critical Public Health* **14**(4): 325–328.

Newbould, J., Taylor, D., Bury, M. (2006) Lay-led self-management in chronic illness: a review of the evidence. *Chronic Illness* **2**(4): 249–261.

Noel, P.H., Larme, A.C., Meyer, J., Marsh, G., Correa, A., Pugh, J.A. (1998) Patient choice in diabetes education curriculum: nutritional versus standard content for type 2 diabetes. *Diabetes Care* **21**: 896–901.

Norris, S.L., Lau, J., Smith, S.J., Schmid, C.H., Engelgau, M.M. (2002) Self-management education for adults with type 2 diabetes: a meta-analysis of the effect on glycemic control. *Diabetes Care* **25**: 1159–1171.

Parchman, M.L., Arambula-Solomon, T.G., Hitchcock Noël, P., Larme, A.C., Pugh, J.C. (2003) Stage of change advancement for diabetes self-management behaviors and glucose control. *Diabetes Educator* **29**(1): 128–134.

Paterson, B.L. (2001) The shifting perspectives model of chronic illness. *Journal of Nursing Scholarship* **33**(1): 21–26.

Paterson, B.L., Russell, C., Thorne, S. (2001) Critical analysis of everyday self-care decision making in chronic illness. *Journal of Advanced Nursing* **35**(3): 335–341.

Pawson, R., Greenhalgh, T., Harvey, G., Walshe, K. (2005) Realist review – a new method of systematic review designed for complex policy interventions. *Journal of Health Services Research and Policy* **10**(S1): 21–34.

Piette, J.D. (2000) Satisfaction with automated telephone disease management calls and its relationship to their use. *Diabetes Educator* **26**(6): 1003–1010.

Raji, A., Gomes, H., Beard, J.O., MacDonald, P., Conlin, P.R. (2002) A randomized trial comparing intensive and passive education in patients with diabetes mellitus. *Archives of Internal Medicine* **162**: 1301–1304.

Roe, G. (2005) Harm reduction as paradigm: is better than bad good enough? The origins of harm reduction. *Critical Public Health* **15**: 243–250.

Rosal, M.C., Olendzki, B., Reed, G.W., Gumieniak, O., Scacron, J., Ockene, I. (2005) Diabetes self-management among low-income Spanish-speaking patients: a pilot study. *Annals of Behavioral Medicine* **29**: 225–235.

Ross, S., Grant, A., Counsell, C., Gillespie, W., Russel, I., Prescott, R. (1999) Barriers to participation in randomised controlled trials: a systematic review. *Journal of Clinical Epidemiology* **52**: 1143–1156.

Sarkadi, A., Rosenqvist, U. (2001) Field test of a group education program for type 2 diabetes: measures and predictors of success on individual and group levels. *Patient Education and Counselling* **44**: 129–139.

Sarkadi, A., Rosenqvist, U. (2004) Experience-based group education in type 2 diabetes. A randomized controlled trial. *Patient Education and Counseling* **53**: 291–298.

Shavers, V.L., Lynch, C.F., Burmeister, L.F. (2002) Racial differences in factors that influence the willingness to participate in medical research studies. *Annals of Epidemiology* **12**: 248–256.

Shibayama, T., Kobayashi, K., Takano, A., Kadowaki, T., Kazuma, K. (2007) Effectiveness of lifestyle counseling by certified expert nurse of Japan for non-insulin-treated diabetic outpatients: a 1-year randomized controlled trial. *Diabetes Research and Clinical Practice* **76**(2): 265–268.

Sigurdardottir, A.K., Jonsdottir, H., Benediktsson, R. (2007) Outcomes of educational interventions in type 2 diabetes: WEKA data-mining analysis. *Patient Education and Counseling* **67**(1–2): 21–31.

Single, E. (1995) Defining harm reduction. *Drug and Alcohol Review* **14**: 287–290.

Skelly, A., Carlson, J., Leeman, J., Holditch-Davis, D., Soward, A. (2005) Symptom-focused management for African American women with type 2 diabetes: a pilot study. *Applied Nursing Research* **18**(4): 213–220.

Skinner, T.C., Carey, M.E., Cradock, S. *et al.* (2006) Diabetes education and self-management for ongoing and newly diagnosed (DESMOND): process modelling of pilot study. *Patient Education and Counseling* **64**(1–3): 369–377.

Steed, L., Lankester, J., Barnard, M., Earle, K., Hurel, S., Newman, S. (2005) Evaluation of the UCL diabetes self-management programme (UCL-DSMP): a randomized controlled trial. *Journal of Health Psychology* **10**(2): 261–276.

Stetson, B.A., Carrico, A.R., Beacham, A.O., Ziegler, C.H., Mokshagundam, S.P. (2006) Feasibility of a pilot intervention targeting self-care behaviors in adults with diabetes mellitus. *Journal of Clinical Psychology in Medical Settings* **13**(3): 239–249.

Tang, T.S., Gillard, M.L., Funnell, M.M. *et al.* (2005) Developing a new generation of ongoing self-management support interventions. *Diabetes Educator* **31**(1): 91–97.

Tatarsky, A. (2003) Harm reduction psychotherapy: extending the reach of traditional substance use treatment. *Journal of Substance Use Treatment* **25**(4): 249–256.

Taylor, D., Bury, M. (2007) Chronic illness, expert patients and care transition. *Sociology of Health and Illness* **29**(1): 27–45.

Thoolen, B., de Ridder, D., Bensing, J., Gorter, K., Rutten, G. (2007a) Who participates in diabetes self-management interventions? *Diabetes Educator* 33(3): 465–474.

Thoolen, B., de Ridder, D., Bensing, J. *et al.* (2007b) Effectiveness of a self-management intervention in patients with screen-detected type 2 diabetes. *Diabetes Care* 30: 2832–2837.

Toobert, D.J., Glasgow, R.E., Strycker, L.A. *et al.* (2003) Biologic and quality-of-life outcomes from the Mediterranean Lifestyle Program: a randomized clinical trial. *Diabetes Care* 26: 2288–2293.

Torgerson, D.J., Klaber-Moffet, J., Russel, I.T. (1996) Patient preferences in randomised trials: threat or opportunity. *Journal of Health Services Research* 1: 194–197.

Two Feathers, J., Kieffer, E.C., Palmisano, G. *et al.* (2005) Racial and ethic approaches to community health (REACH) Detroit partnership: improving diabetes-related outcomes among African American and Latino adults. *American Journal of Public Health* 95(9): 1552–1560.

Uitewaal, P., Bruijnzeels, P., de Hoop, T., Hoes, A., Thomas, S. (2004) Feasibility of diabetes peer education for Turkish type 2 diabetes patients in Dutch general practice. *Patient Education and Counseling* 53: 359–363.

Wang, C.-Y., Chan, S.M.A. (2005) Culturally tailored diabetes education program for Chinese Americans: a pilot study. *Nursing Research* 54(5): 347–353.

Wantland, D.J., Portillo, C.J., Holzemer, W.L., Slaughter, R., McGhee, E.M. (2004) The effectiveness of web-based vs. non-web-based interventions: a meta-analysis of behavioral change outcomes. *Medical Internet Research* 6(4): e40.

Weingarten, S.R., Henning, J.M., Badamgarav, E. *et al.* (2002) Interventions used in disease management programmes for patients with chronic illness – which ones work? Meta-analysis of published reports. *British Medical Journal* 325: 1–8.

Williams, G.C., McGregor, H., Zeldman, A., Freedman, Z. (2005) Promoting glycemic control through diabetes self-management: evaluating a patient activation intervention. *Patient Education and Counseling* 56: 28–34.

Young, B.J., Taylor, J., Friede, T. *et al.* (2005) Pro-active call center treatment support (PACCTS) to improve glucose control in type 2 diabetes. *Diabetes Care* 28(2): 278–282.

7. The Potential of Technology for Providing Social Support to People and Families

David B. Nicholas

Introduction

The use of advanced technology has burgeoned in the delivery of health services over recent decades. Advances in technology-based procedures, the use of eHealth and online supports are examples of the many applications that are currently available in promoting health and providing care to patients. Clearly, there has been widespread effort to harness the potential of technology for improved patient and family outcome. In this chapter, the focus is on the emergence of technology to support patients and their families.

Background

The literature clearly suggests the need for social support in promoting patient and family well-being. Health-based social support is a multidimensional concept comprising of elements of emotional support, education and tangible help. It envelops several theoretical constructs – structure, function and appraisal (Stewart & Lagille 2000). The 'structure' of social support refers to specific sources of support. Support 'functioning' addresses the flow of resources or the provision of support and 'appraisal of support' speaks to the actual availability and delivery of the support. Numerous studies identify the benefits of social support for patients and family members (Goodman 1990; Rounds *et al.* 1991; Meier 1997; Dunham *et al.* 1998; Stewart *et al.* 1998; Ritchie *et al.* 2000); however, support resources may be restrained because of imposed limits on support source, function and availability. As an example, the mandate of providing comprehensive social support may be particularly challenging when patients and their families are geographically distant from centralised health-care services, thereby limiting their access to education and support initiatives. In such an instance, support source and function are present but limits to the availability of that support preclude access.

Moreover, health-care delivery has undergone tremendous shifts in recent decades. As a result of new treatment techniques, pharmaceutical advances and technological gains, the lives of many persons with illness have been extended, creating an increasing population of patients who are providing self-care and/or require care by others, in many cases, family members. Amidst this context of increased care demands, health spending reductions are being realised in many jurisdictions. Health-care professionals are thus challenged to ensure that patients and families have sufficient resources of information and support to manage their own care, particularly pressing given that chronic conditions often require extensive and ongoing home-based care.

The Internet as a health resource

Social support via Internet technology (IT) may mitigate some of the present challenges by offering innovative sources of support and may advance the flow of, and the actual ability for individuals to receive, support. Accessibility, flexibility and utilisation are potentially availed as online networks eliminate geographic and scheduling barriers (Galinsky *et al.* 1997; Nicholas 2003). Increasingly, individuals have Internet knowledge and access to the Internet is available to a growing cohort of the population in Western societies. Given the relatively manageable and decreasing costs of some technology-based innovation (e.g. online networks, website development) and the possibility of reaching many patients, an increasing cadre of health-care programmes have integrated online and other technology-based services within their compendium of patient and family services.

As a result of this shift, specialised health services on the Internet have exponentially increased. This once alternative and 'fringe' resource has emerged as a dominant mechanism for providing education and support to individuals and families affected by illness. Given the mobility and transportation restrictions for many patients, constraints are mitigated and resource availability is markedly improved. By using the Internet, consumers have an arsenal of options in being able to search a health term and draw an array of related information and sources of online support. Accordingly, based on this emerging ability, persons with even very rare conditions are now able to find related information and communicate the same with others sharing similar conditions and challenges.

Many types of Internet-based resources currently exist and are available to consumers. For instance, an American-based international paediatric network, entitled STARBRIGHT World® (SBW) (Bush *et al.* 2002) provides online services for ill children. This online system comprises a broadband interactive network for ill children and offers graphically appealing information, entertainment and peer interaction. Specific features of the network included chatrooms, educational videoconferences and a question-and-answer bulletin board. Hosted chats on specialised conditions are provided, as are links to health resources that have been screened and firewalled against access to the Internet. Ability Online, an international electronic messaging network, provides a safe forum of online peer support for children and adolescents with disabilities (www.ablelink.org; www.abilityonline.org). This network, like many others, employs stringent online safety processes including monitoring and privacy mechanisms such as password protection and encryption software.

Another Internet-based resource offers support to family caregivers of older adults with neurodegenerative disease (Marziali & Donahue 2006). The intervention comprises relevant links and video-conferenced, Internet-mediated and manual-guided education and psychosocial support. Findings from this intervention demonstrate beneficial outcomes for caregivers (Marziali & Donahue 2006), cumulatively supporting the potential for online resources across the lifespan.

Case example: Internet use as a means for promoting well-being among adolescents with diabetes

Providing the necessary psychosocial support and education for adolescents with diabetes is crucial because of daily demands of care and diet control. Children with diabetes require extensive adult support; yet adolescents are increasingly independent. Adolescence is a developmental stage in which individuals typically assume more responsibility for the management of a chronic health condition. Access to information from an online network, particularly given adolescents' affinity to technology, can assist in gaining the necessary skills for self-care (Lowe *et al.* 2005).

Analysis of message boards posted on eight public web-based forums for adolescents with diabetes generated key concerns among these adolescents: life tasks, social support, medical care, gaining information, diabetes management and intrapsychic issues (Ravert *et al.* 2004). In recent years, many online health interventions have been established for adolescents and young adults with diabetes to offer education and support. Iafusco and colleagues, who established a chat line for adolescents with diabetes, found that the majority of concerns discussed addressed health management (Iafusco *et al.* 2000). Support and advice tended to be exchanged in managing anxiety, fears and interpersonal and social relationships. In examining forums and message boards on several websites designed for adolescents with diabetes, day-to-day issues such as mobility, travelling away from home, being active, having a balanced diet, intimate relationships, school issues, potential risks to one's health and typical developmental issues were discussed (Ravert *et al.* 2004; Lowe *et al.* 2005).

Emerging evidence thus suggests that online networks offer adolescents a forum for grappling with key issues associated with diabetes management. Being able to share one's life experiences with a quorum of developmentally similar others who also live with diabetes appeared meaningful and beneficial and was possible through online facilitation. In so doing, an online community emerged as potentially effective in augmenting clinical care and specifically in transitioning adolescents towards independence.

Impact of advanced technology in fostering therapeutic gain: overview of relevant research

The literature, although limited in evaluation studies relative to the volume of existing online resources, identifies the Internet as a viable resource fostering patient and family information and support (Hazzard *et al.* 2002; D'Alessandro *et al.* 2004; Massin *et al.* 2006; Wainstein *et al.* 2006; Nicholas & MacCulloch 2007). Wainstein *et al.* (2006) found that 83% of surveyed families were influenced to ask particular questions in face-to-face interactions with their health-care team based on information found on the Internet, suggesting that information technology influences the attitudes of patients and their families towards health care.

A Cochrane review of Interactive Health Communication Applications (IHCAs) found significant positive effects from the use of web-based interventions. IHCA refers to computer or web-based interventions that combine information along with at least one type of support component, such as decision support or behaviour change support. In a review of 24 randomised controlled trial (RCT) studies, it was found that IHCAs had a significant positive effect on increasing knowledge and social support for users (Murray *et al.* 2005). Recent research suggests that the impact of illness-related websites is enhanced because of the ability to incorporate in-depth information (Beall *et al.* 2002) and opportunity for interaction (Nicholas 2003).

Web-based interventions are found to increase hope and decrease social isolation among caregivers of children with various conditions such as depression (Demaso *et al.* 2006) or physical conditions (Nicholas 2003). Through triadic qualitative interviews (child, caregiver and health provider) Nicholas and MacCulloch (2007) found a wide range of benefits from the utilisation of an online network for children with chronic and life-threatening illness, including social support, coping/personal mastery, communication and education. Fewer hospital visits and less utilisation of medical health-care services are reported as a result of web-based sources of information and support (Gustafson *et al.* 1999; Wagner & Greenlick 2001; Chan *et al.* 2003).

In terms of family members providing care, there is growing evidence that advanced technology interventions provide family caregivers with an environment of nurturance and competence. It is well documented that many caregivers struggle to balance the needs of patients with other demands of daily life (McCubbin *et al.* 1981; Charron-Prochownik 1991; Shulman *et al.* 1991; Butler & Smith 1992; Hamlett *et al.* 1992; Stewart *et al.* 1994; Hanson *et al.* 1995; Thompson & Gustafson 1996; Chaney *et al.* 1997; Holden *et al.* 1997; Harris *et al.* 1999; Nicholas 1999a,b; Charron-Prochownik & Kovacs 2000; Gallant 2003). Increased social support is clearly needed in managing the demanding, sometimes confusing, and routinely shifting requirements of a patient's daily care in the home. Dunham *et al.* (1998) evaluated an online peer support network for young single mothers. The network demonstrated reduced social isolation and participants received emotional, informational and tangible support. Outcomes included increased parental coping and social support over the course of the online network intervention. Nicholas and colleagues implemented an online group targeting isolated fathers of children with spina bifida (Nicholas *et al.* 2005). Outcomes comprised information gain, increased support and decreased illness intrusion. In terms of online content, fathers experienced greater knowledge about resources and care approaches fostering coping. Paternal stress was reduced as was illness intrusion in daily life, and fathers reported appreciating greater connection with others.

In summary, Internet-based social support provides convenience and accessibility in that caregivers can take a virtual break from care, in receiving support, while not needing to leave their home. Given the requirements of care, the need to leave the home for some family caregivers may exclude them from obtaining other forms of support. Also unlike printed forms of information and education, web-based information can be continually updated and shifted according to new advances and preferences of consumers or clinicians.

Patients and caregivers generally appear to benefit from support and information. Online resources are deemed helpful, particularly when they are perceived to be user-friendly, offer ease of access and navigation, have a simplified interface, provide interactivity through online peer support, address cogent worries, needs and questions and convey up to date evidence-based information in a given health area. There is a growing body of literature demonstrating the use and efficacy of online and other advanced technology for augmenting patient and family care and optimising outcomes.

Table 7.1 presents selected examples of technology-based interventions in which outcomes have been evaluated. In this review, the type of technology-based intervention delivered is outlined, as are the target populations, interventional outcomes and the study reference. What appears to emerge from the growing body of outcome-based evidence is that online and other advanced technology-based methods generally promote and augment social support provision. What is not yet well evaluated is the risks incurred by participants and, in particular, by vulnerable populations. Also, further understanding of the nuances, mechanisms and elements of technology-based facilitation that either foster or limit therapeutic gain is yet warranted.

Challenges of Online Support

Despite consistent and increasing reports of benefits from advanced technology for promoting support and education, surprisingly little research attention has been given to the risks and detriments of these methods of service delivery. Clearly, online resources expose potential users to a degree of personal risk, particularly when adequate safeguards are not provided. Cyber abuse is an example of potential hazards if persons exchange personal information over the Internet. Falsified identities and other safety concerns have resulted in heightened monitoring processes (Mann & Stewart 2000); however, there continues to be a pressing need for an ethics and patient/family safety lens in ensuring optimal protection of vulnerable participants. Although gains in technology are anticipated in the future, there is a need for vigilance regarding the potential dangers of these innovations.

Beyond safety concerns, there may be legitimate questions about the credibility of some online information leaving consumers susceptible to confusion,

Table 7.1 Examples of interventions implementing advanced technology and their outcomes

Reference	Type of intervention	Population	Outcomes
Bennett *et al.* (2002)	Tailored message intervention to improve medical compliance (regimen, diet and self-monitoring) using web TV	Elderly women with chronic heart condition	• Enjoyable • Appealing to participants • Feasible for further implementation
Bers *et al.* (2003)	Users interactively design and inhabit a virtual city in real time, i.e. virtually communicate with each other; create characters, spaces and stories • 3D graphical computer environment	Children on haemodialysis, clinical and research staff	• Safe and enjoyable • Contributed to coping • Patients appreciated the ability to communicate with others • Used by children as an escape from reality • Felt safer divulging feelings on Internet • Felt more at ease in communicating • Most discussions not about medical treatment or dialysis • Intervention beneficial both to patients and staff • Fostered positive interactions between patients and their caregivers

Table 7.1 *(cont.)*

Reference	Type of intervention	Population	Outcomes
Calbring *et al.* (2006)	Internet bibliotherapy self-help programme • multi-model treatment website based on CBT • minimal contact with the therapist online • homework assignments for each session reviewed by therapist • prompt advice and feedback given after each session • Internet-based, printable instructions • members invited to post messages in online group discussion • Ten interactive web page modules	Adults with panic disorders	Significant improvement on variables including maladaptive cognitions, bodily interpretation, avoidance, general anxiety and depression • outcomes sustained at 9 month follow-up • findings support Internet interventions such as CBT online (more appropriate and effective for people in isolation or people with agoraphobia and/or panic disorders who are not able to leave their homes and join a face-to-face support system)
Coleman *et al.* (2005)	Health-care provider FAQs module as a part of a patient/family chatroom	Adults with pancreatic cancer and their families	After introduction of FAQs, significant decrease in questions about medical treatment

(cont.)

Table 7.1 *(cont.)*

Reference	Type of intervention	Population	Outcomes
Coulson (2005)	Support network bulletin board • comprises online social support including emotional, self-esteem, networking, tangible assistance and information	Individuals with irritable bowel syndrome (ages not given)	• Active members were very attentive to each other and responded thoroughly to posts in a timely manner • Communication centred around sharing information and support, particularly around medical management, understanding symptoms and navigating the medical world
Dew *et al.* (2004)	Web-based stress and medical management workshops, discussion board, Q and As, links, resources	Adult heart transplant recipients and family caregivers	• Less anxiety, hostility and depression • Greater social functioning and quality of life • Patients used the site more than their caregivers
Glasgow *et al.* (2003)	Web-based information, tailored self-management training and peer support	Novice adult Internet users with type 2 diabetes	• Improvement in dietary, psychosocial and behavioural outcomes • Limited beneficial self-management outcomes

Table 7.1 (*cont.*)

Reference	Type of intervention	Population	Outcomes
Hardey (2002)	Personal web pages (online narratives of persons with illness)	Patients with varying illness (ages not given)	• Express self, provide explanation and support • Advocacy, community organising, information • Narrate daily experience • Meaning making
Hill *et al.* (2006)	Online peer-led asynchronous chat room providing support	Chronically ill women living in rural communities	• Access to support by persons who otherwise may lack access to rural home location • Increase demonstrated in self-esteem, social support and empowerment
Hoffman *et al.* (2001)	Virtual reality distraction helmet with strong sensory input (computer-simulated environment conveying illusion of flying through a virtual environment)	Adults with periodontis	• Eased dental pain during non-surgical procedures (viewed as yet preliminary findings) • Attention drawn away from the real world (e.g. pain)
Holden *et al.* (2002)	Videoconferencing, instant messages, chat rooms, bulletin boards, email, online activities and games, health information	Children with illness	Satisfaction

(*cont.*)

Table 7.1 *(cont.)*

Reference	Type of intervention	Population	Outcomes
Klinger *et al.* (2006)	Virtual supermarket in which patients complete specific tasks in a virtual world that are comparable to daily activities that would be assessed for cognitive function • virtual environment to facilitate assessments of cognitive planning	Adults with Parkinson's disease	Demonstrates the potential of virtual simulation for assessment of real-life events
Kuhl *et al.* (2006)	Varying web-based interventions	Patients with cardiovascular conditions	• Increased patient knowledge, compliance, independence, medical management and quality of life • Associated with positive behavioural, educational, social and financial gain
Marziali *et al.* (2005)	Replication of face-to-face group process through an Internet videoconferencing link • meeting online with a facilitator (social worker or nurse) for weekly group meetings • first 10 weeks professionally	Family caregivers of individuals with neurodegen-erative disease	• Videoconference between participants can mirror a face-to-face group in terms of process, bonding and empathic support • Most group participants reported satisfaction and increased coping

Table 7.1   (*cont.*)

Reference	Type of intervention	Population	Outcomes
	facilitated, after that completely member-run (mutual self-help group) • professionals available as needed (facilitators maintained contact with group via email and phone)		• Members communicated with mutual respect through discussion of the cognitive, emotional and environmental barriers influencing caregiving • Group transition from being professionally moderated to being peer run happened very smoothly
Nicholas (2003)	Chatroom-based mutual aid	Fathers of children with spina bifida	• Decreased isolation and intrusion of illness in daily life • Increased knowledge and coping
Pierce *et al.* (2002)	Weekly online surveys and email discussion	Caregivers of stroke survivors	• Reported satisfaction • Challenges experienced when participants are not knowledgeable about technology • Therapeutic for participants who are receptive to writing experiences; however, less so

(cont.)

Table 7.1   *(cont.)*

Reference	Type of intervention	Population	Outcomes
			for those less comfortable expressing emotion through writing
Rotondi *et al.* (2005)	Interactive web page with information, support and guidance • password protected • online support group • expert Q and A library • resource library • community events	Adults with traumatic brain injuries and their family caregiver	• Website access barriers common to in-person interventions, such as being homebound and lack of transportation • Psychosocial and emotional support services can be effectively provided online
Skinner and Latchford (2006)	E-therapy – refers to any psychological treatment using the Internet	E-therapy users, users of regular Internet mental health support and f2f counselling clients (16–65 years)	• No statistically significant difference in self-disclosure styles between Internet groups and f2f groups (however, there seemed to be a slightly higher tendency to self-disclose in f2f groups) • Those who sought out the Internet mental health groups reported more positive views of E-therapy

Table 7.1 *(cont.)*

Reference	Type of intervention	Population	Outcomes
Whalen *et al.* (2006)	Interactive electronic diary to document daily challenges including interactions, moods, behaviours, social contexts	Children with ADHD and their mothers	• Electronic diaries proved useful for understanding the daily experiences of families in which a child has ADHD • Allows for development of tailored intervention • Applicable for families with little or no chaos

CBT, cognitive behavioural therapy; ADHD, attention-deficit hyperactivity disorder; FAQ, frequently asked questions; Q and A, questions and answers; f2f, face-to-face.

unscrupulous advice and/or harm. There is a need for monitoring of health website information in order to assess for credibility, legitimacy and authorial competence based on best practices. Online information currently appears idiosyncratic, inconsistent and incomplete. In a recent review of social work websites at key paediatric health-care institutions worldwide, only 27% offered psychosocial-based online information and this information was often limited to brief descriptions referencing local services with no links to other sites (Nicholas *et al.* 2005). Accordingly, while advanced technology offers promise in providing or augmenting conventional clinical care, many such resources exist but are not well developed and, in fact, may lack evidence-based content. Apart from greater surveillance and monitoring of online content, there is need for the development of methods and education among health-care providers and lay consumers, addressing how to effectively adjudicate online and other advanced technology-based resources. Efforts have been advanced for assessing online services, comprising criteria rating content, support, interactivity, feedback mechanisms, design and presentation, currency, accessibility, availability, navigation, links and clarity of intended audience (Nicholas & MacCulloch 2007).

Of further concern from a global perspective is the limited evidence of cultural diversity found in online resources (Bomberg *et al.* 1995; Flatley-Brennan 1998; McKay *et al.* 2002; Zarcadoolas *et al.* 2002; Maheu 2003; Nicholas & Mac-Culloch 2007), although emerging data suggests the feasibility of online support for individuals with less literacy and lower socio-economic status as well as culturally diverse populations. Zarcadoolas and colleagues suggest that vulnerable populations exhibit enthusiasm at the prospect of online resources and expect to find online help (Zarcadoolas *et al.* 2002). While the Internet can, to an extent, level the 'playing field' by potentially shielding visible difference, issues of difference and cultural competence remain an issue that has not been sufficiently addressed in virtual applications or the technology-based literature. Concerns arise in that if individuals from minority groups or variant world regions expect relevant help and information on the Internet, they may be more likely to believe and apply for online information and advice, even if spurious, culturally irrelevant or contextually misguided.

The method and type of online application is demonstrated to have an impact upon perceived outcome. In a recent evaluation of online peer support among hospitalised children, a portion of participants reported discomfort in divulging personal information to someone not previously known (Nicholas & MacCulloch 2007). Instances of discomfort were also noted when camera-imaging technology was utilised. While this innovation of video-imaging is reported to reduce isolation, instances of self-consciousness over viewing one's own image online or being seen by others must be considered. Moreover, ethical and informed decision-making is crucial in engaging participants in online activity.

Despite inherent risks, online applications of social support generally appear to be reported as a positive resource, particularly if effectively and ethically managed. Means of controlling risk and promoting safety heighten consideration for safeguards such as participant verification, content monitoring and controlled access to interactivity. As an example, Ability Online utilises traditional mail to ensure that reported names and addresses of users are legitimate. Encryption and password protection are enacted for interactive information. Such safety mechanisms are required and invite careful scrutiny of risks, as well as online competency on the part of service provider personnel. Informed consent and an ethical framework need to be integrated in order to ensure due diligence for safety promotion. Participants need to be educated about the potential benefits of the resource as well as the risks and safeguards of online interventions in order to make an informed choice about involvement. Vulnerable populations may require enhanced safety guidelines and mechanisms in optimising their protection and upholding their rights. Application of an ethical lens to decision-making is urgently warranted regarding the use of advanced technology for clinical and research use. This seems particularly cogent when considering applications with paediatric, disabled, geriatric and other vulnerable populations.

Social support delivery: considerations in selecting advanced technology methods

In our review of literature addressing advanced technology-based applications, positive outcomes are largely identified with less consideration of how and under what conditions online applications yield desirable (or conversely, less desirable) outcomes. Towards best practices in online social support provision, programme planners and clinicians must consider interventional aims, characteristics of the target population, communication preferences, accessibility of the online method offered, availability of the population to actually use the intervention (e.g. family caregivers may have access to computers but lack time to engage in an online intervention) and population affinity to online capacities. As an example of population affinity, computer-savvy adolescents may be more likely to participate in an online network than in a face-to-face group. Working fathers of chronically ill children, who necessarily miss clinical support sessions due to work commitments, may similarly be more likely to engage in online support.

Into the virtual future . . .

Optimal methods for facilitating helpful information and support through advanced technology will vary over time and according to targeted populations and aims. Clearly, there is a growing trend towards portability and integration of technology as biological, physiological, care management and support aims can increasingly intersect through advancing cellular and micro-technology. Computer screens may increasingly give way to cell phones and palm-sized portable devices, providing full access to the Internet and other advanced technology sources. Variant strands of technology mediation will no doubt emerge in directions not yet envisaged. A recent example is the proliferation of advanced technology for the delivery of graduate education. Education and support to patients, families and health-care providers, including inter-professional health-based students, will likely markedly advance both in academia and practice settings. Accordingly, best practices can be examined and disseminated through network-generated, evidence-based online approaches. Virtual and cascaded fact sheets and webcast seminars conveying best practice strategies for optimal patient care can be promoted and mass delivered through technology access.

Anticipating future directions is an unknown art in part because technology and its future capacities are moving targets that are largely unbridled and hence difficult to regulate or control. Regardless of the course of this development, it appears safe to assume that there will be continued virtual access and widespread utilisation within the health-care service delivery. Towards this end, monitoring, patient safety and regulatory review are pressing needs as online potentialities rapidly shift and may be more or less effective for varying clinical contexts and among particular populations. Health-care professionals cannot relegate technology-mediated health content solely to the scrutiny of IT colleagues or the general public in their consumption of publicly accessible health information and support. Instead, it seems crucial that new inter-professional, multisectoral models be developed and tested for the optimal delivery, monitoring, updating and best practices in health practice delivery via advanced technology.

Clearly, we are at a precipice in which advanced technology is increasingly integral and viable within the delivery of health care. Technology transcends what might appear to be the mere 'point and click of the mouse' as online capacities point towards meaningful support, greater health knowledge and better patient outcomes. However, while riding this wave of technology transformation we are well advised not to lose sight of prudence as we uphold patient and family safety and ensure an ethical integration of innovation and technology.

References

Beall, M.S., Golladay, G.J., Greenfield, M.V., Hensinger, R.N., Beirmann, J.S. (2002) Use of Internet by orthopaedic outpatients. *Journal of Pediatric Orthopaedics* **22**: 261–264.

Bennett, S.J., Hays, L.M., Embree, J.L., Arnould, M. (2002) Heart messages: a tailored message intervention for improving heart failure outcomes. *The Journal of Cardiovascular Nursing* **14**(4): 94–105.

Bers, M.U., Gonzalez-Heydrich, J., DeMaso, D.R. (2003) Use of a computer-based application in a pediatric hemodialysis unit: a pilot study. *Journal of the American Academy of Child and Adolescent Psychiatry* **24**(4): 493–496.

Bomberg, E.W., Gustafson, D.H., Hawkins, R.P. *et al.* (1995) Development, acceptance, and use patterns of a computer-based education and social support system for people living with AIDS/HIV infection. *Computers in Human Behavior* **11**(2): 289–311.

Bush, J.P., Huchital, J.R., Simonian, S.J. (2002) An introduction to program and research initiatives of the STARBRIGHT foundation. *Children's Health Care* **31**(1): 1–10.

Butler, S., Smith, D. (1992) Living with chronic pediatric liver disease: the parent's experience. *Pediatric Nursing* **18**(5): 236–247.

Calbring, P., Bohman, S., Brunt, S. *et al.* (2006) Remote treatment of panic disorder: a randomized trial of Internet based cognitive behavior therapy supplemented with telephone calls. *The American Journal of Psychiatry* **163**(12): 2119–2125.

Chan, D.S., Callahan, C.W., Sheets, S.J., Moreno, C.N., Malone, F.J. (2003) An Internet-based store-and-forward video home telehealth system for improving asthma outcomes in children. *American Journal of Health System Pharmacy* **60**: 1976–1981.

Chaney, J.M., Mullins, L.L., Frank, R.G. *et al.* (1997) Transactional patterns of child, mother, and father adjustment in insulin-dependent diabetes mellitus: a prospective study. *Journal of Pediatric Psychology* **22**(2): 229–244.

Charron-Prochownik, D. (1991) *Social Support, Chronic Stress, and Health Outcomes in Adolescents with Diabetes*. University of Michigan: Ann Arbour, MI.

Charron-Prochownik, D., Kovacs, M. (2000) Maternal health-related coping patterns and health and adjustment outcomes in children with type 1 diabetes. *Children's Health Care* **29**(1): 37–45.

Coleman, J., Olsen, S.J., Sauter, P.K. *et al.* (2005) The effect of a frequently asked questions module on a pancreatic cancer web site patient/family chat room. *Cancer Nursing* **28**(6): 460–468.

Coulson, N. (2005) Receiving social support online: an analysis of a computer-mediated support group for individuals living with irritable bowel syndrome. *Cyberpsychology and Behavior* **8**(6): 580–584.

D'Alessandro, D., Kreiter, C.D., Kinzer, K.L., Peterson, M.W. (2004) A randomized controlled trial of information prescription for pediatric patient education on the Internet. *Archives of Pediatrics and Adolescent Medicine* **158**: 857–862.

Demaso, D.R., Marcus, N.E., Kinnamon, C., Gonzalez-Heydrich, J. (2006) Depression experience journal: a computer-based intervention for families facing childhood depression. *American Academy of Child and Adolescent Psychiatry* **45**(2): 158–165.

Dew, M.A., Goycoolea, J.M., Harris, R.C. *et al.* (2004) An Internet based intervention to improve psychosocial outcomes in heart transplant recipients and family caregivers: development and evaluation. *Journal of Heart and Lung Transplantation* 23: 745–758.

Dunham, P.J., Hurshman, A., Litwin, E., Gusella, J., Ellsworth, C., Dodd, P.W. (1998) Computer-mediated social support: single young mothers as a model system. *American Journal of Community Psychology* 26: 281–306.

Flatley-Brennan, P. (1998) Computer network home care demonstration: a randomized trial in persons living with AIDS. *Computers in Biology and Medicine* 28: 489–508.

Galinsky, M.J., Schopler, J.H., Abell, M.D. (1997) Connecting group members through telephone and computer groups. *Health and Social Work* 22: 181–188.

Gallant, M.P. (2003) The influence of social support on chronic illness self-management: a review and directions for research. *Health Education and Behavior* 30(2): 170–195.

Glasgow, R.E., Boles, S.M., McKay, G., Feil, E.G., Barrera, M. (2003) The D-Net diabetes self management program: long-term implementation, outcomes, and generalization results. *Preventive Medicine* 36: 410–419.

Goodman, C. (1990) Evaluation of a model self-help telephone program: impact on natural networks. *Social Work with Groups* 35: 556–562.

Gustafson, D.H., Hawkins, R., Boberg, E. *et al.* (1999) Impact of a patient-centred, computer-based health information/support system. *American Journal of Preventive Medicine* 16(1): 1–9.

Hamlett, K.W., Pelligrini, D.S., Katz, K.S. (1992) Childhood chronic illness as a family stressor. *Journal of Pediatric Psychology* 17(1): 33–47.

Hanson, C.L., De Guire, M.J., Schinkel, A.M., Kolterman, O.G. (1995) Empirical validation for a family-centered model of care. *Diabetes Care* 18: 1347–1356.

Hardey, M. (2002) The story of my illness: personal accounts of illness on the Internet. *Health: An Interdisciplinary Journal for the Social Study of Health, Illness, and Medicine* 6(1): 31–46.

Harris, M.A., Greco, P., Wysocki, T., Elder-Danda, C., White, N.H. (1999) Adolescents with diabetes from single-parent, blended and intact families: health-related and family functioning. *Families, Systems and Health* 17(2): 181–196.

Hazzard, A., Celkano, M., Collins, M., Markov, Y. (2002) Effects of STARBRIGHT world on knowledge, social support and coping in hospitalized children with sickle cell disease and asthma. *Children's Health Care* 31(1): 69–86.

Hill, W., Weinert, C., Cudney, S. (2006) Influence of a computer intervention on the psychological status of chronically ill rural women. *Nursing Research* 55(1): 34–42.

Hoffman, H.C., Garcia-Palacios, A., Patterson, D.R., Jensen, M., Furness, T., Ammons, W.P. (2001) The effectiveness of virtual reality for dental pain control: a case study. *Cyberpsychology and Behavior* 4(4): 527–535.

Holden, E.W., Chmielewski, D., Nelson, C.C., Kager, V.A., Foltz, L. (1997) Controlling for general and disease-specific effects in child and family adjustment to chronic childhood illness. *Journal of Pediatric Psychology* 22(1): 15–27.

Holden, G., Bearison, D.J., Rode, D.C., Kapiloff, M.F., Rosenberg, G., Rosenzweig, J. (2002) The impact of a computer network on pediatric pain and anxiety: a randomized control clinical trial. *Social Work in Health Care* 36(2): 21–33.

Iafusco, D., Ingenito, N., Prisco, F. (2000) The chatline as a communication and educational tool in adolescents with insulin-dependent diabetes: preliminary observations. *Diabetes Care* 23(12): 1853.

Klinger, E., Chemin, I., Lebreton, S., Marie, R.M. (2006) Virtual action planning in Parkinson's disease: a control study. *Cyberpsychology and Behavior* 9(3): 342–347.

Kuhl, E.A., Sears, S.F., Conti, J.B. (2006) Internet-based behavioral change and psychosocial care for patients with cardiovascular disease: a review of cardiac disease specific applications. *Heart and Lung* 35: 374–382.

Lowe, P., Hearnshaw, H., Griffiths, F. (2005) Attitudes of young people with diabetes to an Internet-based virtual clinic. *Journal of Telemedicine and Telecare* 11 (Suppl 1): 59–60.

Maheu, M.M. (2003) The online clinical management model. *Psychotherapy: Theory, Research, Practice, Training* 40(1/2): 20–32.

Mann, C., Stewart, F. (2000) *Internet Communication and Qualitative Research*. Sage Publication: Thousand Oaks, CA.

Marziali, E., Donahue, P. (2006) Caring for others: Internet video-conferencing group intervention for family caregivers of older adults with neurodegenerative disease. *The Gerontologist* 46(3): 398–403.

Marziali, E., Donahue, P., Crossin, G. (2005) Caring for others: Internet health care support intervention for family caregivers of persons with Alzheimer's, stroke, or Parkinson's disease. *Families in Society* 86(3): 375–383.

Massin, M.M., Montesanti, J., Gerard, P. (2006) Use of the Internet by parents of children with congenital heart disease. *Acta Cardiologica* 61(1): 406–410.

McCubbin, H.I., McCubbin, M.A., Nevin, R., Cauble, A.E. (1981) Coping health inventory for parents (CHIP). In: McCubbin, H.I., Thompson, A.I., McCubbin, M.A. (eds) *Family Assessment: Resiliency, Coping and Adaptation – Inventories for Research and Practice*. University of Wisconsin System: Madison, WI.

McKay, H.G., Glasgow, R.E., Feil, E.G., Boles, S.M., Barrera, M. (2002) Internet-based diabetes self-management and support: initial outcomes from the diabetes network project. *Rehabilitation Psychology* 47(1): 31–48.

Meier, A. (1997) Inventing new models of social support groups: a feasibility study of an online stress management support group for social workers. *Social Work with Groups* 20(4): 35–53.

Murray, E., Burns, J., See Tai, S., Lai, R., Nazareth, I. (2005) Interactive health communications applications for people with chronic disease. *Cochrane Database of Systematic Reviews* Issue 4: Art. No.: CD004274. DOI: 10.1002/14651858.CD004274.pub4.

Nicholas, D.B. (1999a) The lived experience of mothers caring for a child with end stage renal disease. *Qualitative Health Journal* 9(A): 468–478.

Nicholas, D.B. (1999b) Meanings of maternal caregiving: children with end stage renal disease. *Qualitative Health Research* 9(4): 468–478.

Nicholas, D.B. (2003) Participant perceptions of online groupwork with fathers of children with spina bifida. In: Sullivan, N., Mesbur, E.S., Lang, N.C., Goodman, D., Mitchell, L. (eds) *Social Work with Groups: Social Justice through Personal, Community, and Societal Change*. The Haworth Press, Inc.: Binghamton, NY, pp. 227–240.

Nicholas, D.B., MacCulloch, R. (2007) *An Examination of Cross Cultural Issues in Online Support*.

Nicholas, D.B., McNeill, T., Antle, B.J. (2005) *Review of Psychosocial Websites*. Hospital for Sick Children: Toronto, ON.

Pierce, L., Steiner, V., Govoni, A.L. (2002) In-home online support for caregivers of survivors of stroke: a feasibility study. *Computers, Informatics, Nursing* 20(4): 1538–2931.

Ravert, R., Hancock, M., Ingersoll, G. (2004) Online forum messages posted by adolescents with type 1 diabetes. *Diabetes Educator* **30**(5): 827–834.

Ritchie, J.A., Stewart, M.J., Ellerton, M.L. *et al.* (2000) Parents' perceptions of the impact of a telephone support group intervention. *Journal of Family Nursing* **6**: 25–45.

Rotondi, A.J., Sinkule, J., Spring, M. (2005) An interactive web based intervention for persons with TBI and their families. Use and evaluation by female significant others. *The Journal of Head Trauma Rehabilitation* **20**(2): 173–185.

Rounds, K.A., Galinsky, M.F., Stevens, L.S. (1991) Linking people with AIDS in rural communities: the telephone group. *Social Work* **36**: 13–18.

Shulman, S., Fisch, R.O., Zempel, C.E., Gadish, O., Chang, P.N. (1991) Children with phenylketonuria: the interface of family and child functioning. *Journal of Developmental and Behavioral Pediatrics* **12**(5): 315–321.

Skinner, A.E.G., Latchford, G. (2006) Attitudes to counseling via the Internet: a comparison between in-person counseling clients and Internet support group users. *Counseling and Psychotherapy Research* **6**(3): 158–163.

Stewart, M.J., Doble, S., Hart, G., Langille, L., MacPherson, K. (1998) Peer visitor support for family caregivers of seniors with stroke. *Canadian Journal of Nursing Research* **30**: 87–117.

Stewart, M.J., Lagille, L. (2000) *A Framework for Social Support Assessment and Intervention in the Context of Chronic Conditions and Caregiving*. University of Toronto Press: Toronto, ON.

Stewart, M.J., Ritchie, J.A., McGrath, P., Thompson, D., Bruce, B. (1994) Mothers of children with chronic conditions: supportive and stressful interactions with partners and professionals regarding caregiving burdens. *Canadian Journal of Nursing Research* **26**(4): 61–82.

Thompson, R.J., Gustafson, K.E. (1996) *Adaptation to Chronic Childhood Illness*. American Psychological Association: Washington, DC.

Wagner, T.H., Greenlick, M.R. (2001) When parents are given greater access to health information, does it affect pediatric utilization? *Medical Care* **39**(8): 848–855.

Wainstein, B.K., Sterling-Levis, K., Baker, S.A., Taitz, J., Brydon, M. (2006) Use of Internet by parents of paediatric patients. *Journal of Paediatrics and Child Health* **42**: 528–532.

Whalen, C.K., Henker, B., Jamner, L.D. *et al.* (2006) Toward mapping daily challenges of living with ADHD: maternal and child perspectives using electronic diaries. *Journal of Abnormal Child Psychology* **34**(1): 115–130.

Zarcadoolas, C., Blanco, M., Boyer, J.F., Pleasant, A. (2002) Unweaving the web: an exploratory study of low-literate adults' navigation skills on the world wide web. *Journal of Health Communication* **7**: 309–324.

8. *Chronic Illness Research: Translating What We Know into What We Do*

*Renee F. Lyons, Lynn McIntyre, Grace Warner,
Celeste Alvaro, Alastair Buchan, Ian Reckless
and Alison Kitson*

Introduction

Global health statistics provide a relatively clear picture about projected chronic illness prevalence and its impact over the next 25–30 years. The picture is not pretty. Correspondingly, health policy analyses, irrespective of the country, consistently report that current efforts to address chronic illnesses are inadequate despite considerable clinical and population health knowledge about actions that would substantially improve prevention, management and quality of life. It is incumbent upon our generation to provide improved leadership in clarifying chronic illness prevalence and its determinants and launching major initiatives to address it.

Research is an important key to unlocking solutions to the growing burden of chronic illness, but only if society is prepared to use quality evidence in decision-making. Billions of dollars are spent on creating evidence. We now need more investment and know-how in applying quality evidence to societal problems such as chronic illness. So, instead of focusing directly on the obvious value of generating more knowledge about health and illness, this chapter speaks of how we might positively modify future projections of chronic illness by building upon the revolution that is happening in some parts of the globe in knowledge translation.

Knowledge translation (KT) is about the process of using research in decision-making. It integrates elements of knowledge generation (what we study and how), exchange (communication between researchers and users) and use (changes to current thought, practice and/or policy). Kitsons' Promoting Action on Research Implementation in Health Services framework (PARiHS) is offered as a guide for considering how research can be mobilised more effectively to advance KT for chronic illness prevention and treatment.

We take a somewhat macroscopic approach to both KT and the PARiHS framework. Individual pieces of evidence that translate into improved practice are vitally important. However, KT needs a supportive environment for applying knowledge – an environment that engages people (e.g. planners and policymakers, clinicians, citizens, students, researchers) in a positive way at all levels in finding solutions to chronic illness. It requires bold government leadership and adequate infrastructure to substantially increase and speed up the use of high-quality evidence and practice guidelines within health systems. In other words, improvements in knowledge use can be advanced through a whole systems perspective that moves countries (and collections of countries) and their citizens towards application of evidence in achieving specific goals in the fight against chronic illness – a chronic illness social movement of sorts. Stroke is used as a case study at different points in the chapter.

The task ahead

The gift of longevity has guaranteed a prominent place for chronic illness, now and into the future. The number of people over 80 years of age in Western Europe, for instance, has quadrupled in 60 years (Watkins 2004). Living longer, together with improved health maintenance and restorative services means that most of us will live with some sort of chronic illness in our lifetime and particularly in our older years. Add to these 'gifts' society's resistance to substantively address modifiable personal and population risk factors such as poor-quality food, inactivity, environmental contaminants, poverty and health disparity, and we are heading into a challenging (albeit highly modifiable) health trajectory.

Chronic illness is currently the main cause of both death and disability worldwide. Of the 58 million deaths that occurred in 2005, approximately 35 million, or 60%, were due to chronic causes, primarily cardiovascular disease, diabetes, cancer and respiratory conditions (Abegunde *et al*. 2007). Despite some recent reduction in mortality rates associated with cardiovascular disease, future projections are discouraging. In 2030, chronic illness is predicted to cause three quarters of all deaths (WHO 2008). In the United States, 7 out of every 10 deaths are caused by chronic illness, and health-care spending on people with chronic conditions is projected to double between 2000 and 2010 (Zhang *et al*. 2001).

Morbidity and co-morbidities are also on the rise with population ageing, especially in the Western world. In the United Kingdom, for instance, 80% of general practitioner consultations are related to chronic illness. And of the 17 million people currently living with long-term conditions in the United Kingdom, up to 80% need support for self-care (DH 2004). The number of people with disabilities in the United States is large and growing: 49.7 million non-institutionalised people report disabilities and about 21.5 million of these are working-age adults (U.S. Census Bureau 2003).

The social and economic costs of chronic illness are enormous. For instance, calculations of the total economic burden of seven types of the most prevalent chronic illnesses (medical costs and productivity loss) in Canada exceed $93 billion a year (Chronic Disease Prevention Alliance of Canada 2004).

Those in the most disadvantaged socio-economic groups experience the highest chronic illness prevalence and mortality rates, and the gap in health inequalities has been widening (Crombie *et al.* 2005). Although there has been considerable knowledge gained in understanding health disparities and their determinants, action has been slow (Reich *et al.* 2008). The results of numerous countrywide policies to reduce health disparities have not been encouraging and there is recognition by some governments (e.g. England) that reversing the trends in health disparities will require focused and sustained inter-sectoral collaborations at national and local levels over time as measured in generations (DH 2006; Keon 2008).

Although there is an increased clarity on some fronts regarding the growing problem of chronic illness, there are many uncertainties about what sort of future to expect. For instance, most demographers who study ageing and health include accommodation in their predictions for many possible future scenarios (Harper 2006). What are the limits of longevity? How will potential changes in social and physical environments (e.g. poverty, global warming) impact chronic illness? Also, there is little clarity about how the health of current generations has been influenced by gene–environment interactions experienced in past generations. If we were to substantively reduce population health risk factors today, how would they affect chronic illnesses prevalence? Some bio-demographers suggest that because the prevalence of chronic disease is primarily among older adults, the general effects of ageing combined with chronic illness will require major intervention to produce positive gains (Carnes & Olshansky 2007).

Despite some questions about the future of chronic illness and ageing, there is considerable evidence of the need to act (i.e. analyses of quality of care and illness burden and advances in prevention and management). There is also agreement between many health leaders that the challenges for society, now and into the future, are how to prevent illness, how to compress morbidity so that we live more disability-free years and how to reduce the preventable, devastating effects of illness, including delay of onset, recurrence and burden (Choi *et al.* 2008). The following action list, which combines social and health elements, would be a good start in addressing these challenges:

- Risk factor reduction and improvement in the social and physical environments that contribute to illness and injury, such as poverty
- Advances in effective and cost-effective clinical approaches, which encompass risk assessment and management
- Integrated health care for individuals and their families, which includes guidance and support for health socialisation
- Action to reduce the heavy burden of care-giving of chronically ill and disabled dependents

- Increases in applied clinical, prevention and population health intervention research
- Bold new ways to apply research evidence in health-related decision-making at all levels
- Special attention to middle and low resource regions and to health disparities.

Similar lists of chronic illness strategies have been replicated around the world. Likewise, people sit together in planning sessions not infrequently at regional, national and international gatherings, to plot frameworks and approaches to address these issues. The task is daunting as major issues must be addressed if we are to transform policy and practice.

Complex problems such as chronic illness require comprehensive, high-level strategic investments, as well as practical action within and across all health-related sectors. We need to ask about the dose–response required to substantively impact health outcomes and where we should place our efforts. Are we thinking boldly and strategically? What are the interventions at a clinical and population level that will truly impact the ever-growing burden of disease? In many cases we know what to do. What is holding us back? There appears to be considerable paralysis in the abilities and willingness of many nations to act.

The dose–response problem

As with the challenges of climate change and global warming, data and experience indicate that we are touching the edges of a tsunami-size chronic illness wave. Among health professionals and the public, there is a feeling, backed by evidence, that what is being done to address chronic illness (despite contributing valuable pieces of the health puzzle) is simply fragmented and inadequate. Although chronic illness is not usually considered communicable by traditional definitions, the global socialisation to risk factors such as smoking, unhealthy dietary habits and inactivity could be considered communicable in the social sense (Choi *et al.* 2008). Dose–response, in this context, means that a big problem such as chronic illness needs a strategically developed attack plan of considerable dimension in order to make a difference.

How are people thinking about this issue? Many people worldwide have been studying the problem of chronic illness and what we should do about it. An informal Internet search of the term 'chronic illness' together with 'the future of' resulted in over 1.8 million documents that speak of some aspect of the issue. Included are a plethora of research, personal accounts, guidelines and policy directives. These websites proffer issues, strategies and products focused on the full range of individual, family, health systems or population health issues.

Agency websites provide interpretations of the problem of chronic illness and approaches to prevention and management; for example, the Robert Wood Johnson Commission (US) (www.rwjf.org) looks beyond the medical care system to the social determinants of health differences; the Province of Ontario, Canada, establishes a Department of Health Protection and Promotion (www.health.gov.on.ca)

166

and the National Health Service (Britain) launches its new obesity, vascular checks and stroke strategies (www.dh.gov.uk). Despite this flurry of activity, concerted action by countries, even highly resourced countries, varies considerably.

Why is it that some countries are moving boldly forward in chronic disease prevention and management, and others are not? Critiquing Canada's inaction on the documented promises of substantive health system reforms, Lewis (2007) comments:

> *Canada's apparent capacity to reform its health system is inversely proportionate to the volume of high quality reports that document the need to do so. . . . . The connection between intention and action seems stronger and more immediate elsewhere. Other countries aren't Nirvana, but their errors are braver – sins of commission than omission . . . They think, they plan, they act, often decisively. Somehow the risks of innovation and policy experimentation seem lower. They are less afraid to set meaningful targets and shoot at them. . . . . The United Kingdom exhausts its system with perpetual change; we exhaust ours with endless talk and death by a thousand demonstration projects.*

Bringewatt (2003), speaking on behalf of the National Chronic Care Consortium in the United States, echoes these views. He suggests that in the United States, market forces continue to reinforce an outdated approach to serving people with chronic illness and disability, health care's largest, highest cost and fastest growing service group. He urges people to rise above their immediate short-term self-interest and recognise the interdependence of their decision-making. Long-term systems-oriented approaches shaped by the nature of chronic illness rather than the antiquated structures on which programmes were established are needed – and needed now.

Overall, the clear take-home message is that efforts to address the growing burden of chronic illness in most countries suffer from the dose–response problem. A more aggressive approach to prevention and management through population health and health systems reforms is needed. The future of chronic illness will depend on agreement on how to approach, prioritise and distribute resources. The future will also depend on how we clarify and address tensions that cause resistance to formulating a strong change agenda – tensions including economics vs. health, prevention vs. treatment, acute vs. chronic, chronic disease vs. illness-specific approaches, population health vs. individual health, need vs. evidence, screening vs. case-finding, community-based vs. institutions. A simple example is the resistance to create walking- and bike-friendly communities in the face of rising obesity rates, climate change and the price of fuel. Such changes inconvenience cars, their makers and users.

The lack of attention from researchers and policymakers to population-based prevention, given its potential in reducing the incidence of chronic illness, will likely be a major focus for the future. 'Health for All' policies are emerging as mechanisms to draw governments to use a population health lens across government departments. South Australia is an example of a region that has developed a set of core principles that will influence policy decisions from a health perspective. Given the promise of a substantive dose–response using this approach, South Australia will be an important natural experiment to watch in examining whether this policy lens approach can effect government policy change and impact the rate of chronic illness in the region (Kickbusch *et al.* 2008).

Chronic illness is undeniably complex, and barriers to the uptake of evidence and innovation are more difficult in complex circumstances (Landry *et al.* 2002). However, it is becoming easier, through advances in global health statistics and monitoring, to demonstrate some clear problem areas and potential wins in the fight for chronic illness prevention. If tobacco is a risk factor for six out of the eight leading causes of death, results in almost 10% of deaths worldwide and the death rates from smoking are expected to rise from 5.4 million in 2004 to 8.3 million in 2030, then this is a substantial area to target. More than 80% of these deaths will be in low- and middle-income countries and efforts to control tobacco currently reach only about 5% of the world's population (WHO 2008). Attributions for why so many people are still smoking could be made to its addictive properties. However, market forces, especially in these countries, may be the greatest contributor.

The promise of research

The theme of this book, 'research into practice', suggests that knowledge and evidence play critically important roles in shaping the action agenda and in addressing chronic illness. Scientists have spent decades conducting research on the mélange of chronic illness prevention and treatment themes and many of these research advances have been described throughout the book, for example, e-health (see Chapter 7). Research has taken us a lot further in understanding and acting on population, genetic and clinical determinants of health and illness than could have been imagined 50 or even 10 years ago.

Although there remain numerous unanswered questions, controversies, contradictions and critiques for most health questions, research has drawn special attention to the issue of chronic illness. It has provided greater clarity about illness prevalence and impact and predictions about what might be expected in the future epidemic of chronic illness. Research also has resulted in numerous theories, tools and strategies for prevention and treatment, including clinical and population approaches to improving care and reducing health disparities. Evidence is becoming a core element in health and policy decisions, and it is these countrywide and international 'movements' that we need to monitor and influence.

Choi *et al.* (2008) state that global health is everyone's concern; yet chronic illness, the leading cause of adult mortality in all countries (Yach *et al.* 2005), has not secured a prominent place on the global health agenda. These authors developed seven themes to consider and build upon in order to enhance future global capacity in surveillance, prevention and control of chronic diseases. The acronym,

SCIENCE, includes the seven themes of **S**trategy, **C**ollaboration, **I**nformation, **E**ducation, **N**ovelty, **C**ommunication and **E**valuation. The idea is to use research and evidence as the basis for decision-making.

Research holds the promise of a bright future for chronic illness prevention and treatment. However, the non-use of evidence and the turtle-like pace of uptake could be considered an important human rights issue. A recent text on the history of cancer systematically documents the development of cancer research and how the lag in research use internationally has resulted in immense social and economic costs (Davis 2007). The same could be said for most chronic illnesses including diabetes (American Diabetes Association 2006) or environmentally caused asthma (Prescott *et al.* 2000). There appears to be an amazing tolerance for lack of research uptake – for inaction that appears scandalous – given the promise of prevention and treatment.

Researchers are working like 'busy bees' researching, publishing and advocating for action; yet very few changes in recent years have occurred that have led to major improvements in prevention and treatment of chronic illness relative to research output (Woolf 2006; Lyons & McIntyre 2007). Why does this busy work not lead to new and more effective policies, that is, policy transforming? If it gets to policy, why does it not make it to practice? Is it that good evidence in many areas of chronic disease prevention and treatment is being ignored? Is it that researchers are poor knowledge translators? Are the investments in research tolerable but investments that would be required for genuine health improvements intolerable? Despite the current attention paid to accountability and outcome research is grossly underused. There is substantial skepticism about evidence and resistance to changing established practice, be it at the individual or health system level. There are also under-developed mechanisms to support research use which, for most types of evidence, is quite difficult – actually, notoriously difficult (Dopson & Fitzgerald 2005).

Kerner (2006) has stated that billions of US tax dollars are spent on basic discovery, intervention development and efficacy research. Billions of US tax dollars are also spent on health service delivery programmes. Little is spent on how to ensure that the lessons learned from science inform and improve the quality of health services and the availability of evidence-based approaches. To close this discovery–delivery gap, researchers and their funding agencies must recognise the gap between basic discovery and intervention development and work together with practitioners and their funding agencies to recognise the growing gap between innovative interventions developed through research and what is actually delivered to reduce the burden of chronic disease.

In order to overcome what Lewis (2007) calls our 'innovation learning disability', major shifts in research, health policy and the linkages between them are needed. To achieve these shifts, researchers must come to grips with how we address personal, institutional and societal challenges in moving research to action. From a clinical and policy perspective, we need to revolutionise how chronic illness prevention and treatment are managed, if we are to effectively use knowledge. And in such KT activities, clarity about how to address broader economic, political and social tensions such as those mentioned earlier is central. Translating lessons learned from science to public health, primary care or disease speciality service settings also require multifaceted collaboration to accelerate the translation of research into practice.

How do we capitalise upon the undeveloped promise for moving research into action? Fortunately, there is much that we can build from in the new approaches being developed in KT research and practice. And there is new energy building to collaborate and to share approaches and responsibility for improvement in KT across the divides: countries, academe, public and private sectors and the voluntary sector (Gibbons 1999; Kitson & Bisby 2008).

Knowledge translation: emerging from naïveté

> *Sometimes the step from best evidence to best practice is simple; however, most of the time it is not ....*
> *(Grol & Grimshaw 2003)*

Research alone does little to effect policy and practice. There is also substantial evidence that traditional mechanisms (e.g. research papers, 10-minute conference presentations, 2-hour evening continuing medical education sessions) used to communicate evidence and best practice result in limited uptake despite strong evidence of the efficacy of the specific innovation for improving practice and policy (Lavis *et al.* 2002; Grol & Grimshaw 2003).

Knowledge translation is the term used by the Canadian Institutes of Health Research (CIHR) to describe the process of putting research findings and products into the hands of key audiences.

> *Knowledge translation is a dynamic and iterative process that includes synthesis, dissemination, exchange and ethically sound application of knowledge to improve the health of Canadians, provide more effective health services and products and strengthen the health-care system. This process takes place within a complex system of interactions between researchers and knowledge users which may vary in intensity, complexity and level of engagement depending on the nature of the research and the findings as well as the needs of the particular knowledge user*
> *(Canadian Institutes of Health Research [CIHR] 2008).*

Implicit in the CIHR definition is the notion that evaluation and monitoring of KT initiatives, processes and activities are key components of the KT process. The move to a KT approach resulted from the demands for increased accountability in research funding. It also evolved as a marketing tool to acquire additional research dollars (e.g. health research will improve health) and from concerns that important research was not being used or was not being taken up quickly enough (Kitson & Bisby 2008).

Chronic Illness Research: Translating What We Know into What We Do

Over the past 10 years, researchers, governments and granting agencies have begun to address these issues through fostering innovation in research synthesis and communication. In fact, one of the greatest single changes in health research and policy development has been the attention paid to KT

(Graham & Tetroe 2007).

Examples of KT functions

Examples of KT functions for knowledge development, exchange and use include the following:

- Research syntheses and evidence-based practice guidelines
- Communication of research results, syntheses and evidence-based practice guidelines
- Forums and symposia that bring together researchers and research users to examine and debate evidence and its application
- Knowledge networks, communities of practice and brokers who facilitate knowledge use
- Development and testing of innovations in communication and knowledge use facilitation (e.g. web-based decision tools)
- Focus groups and committees to identify research needs (generate applied health research questions) and to strategise about how to overcome constraints to knowledge use
- Training in KT for researchers, practitioners, administrators and policymakers
- The use of entertainment education (Singhal *et al.* 2004) such as embedding knowledge fragments in public communication
- Contextualising evidence for/with specific populations and settings
- KT demonstration projects and case study development (Dopson & Fitzgerald 2005)
- Monitoring and evaluation of research uptake
- Studying the effectiveness of KT strategies with respect to institutional and health outcomes

Knowledge translation is evolving as both a practice and a developing science. For instance, KT research in chronic illness can range from the use of behavioural theory in clinician's practice change (Grimshaw 2007), to studies that examine the research's use capacity in health and social systems (Alvaro *et al.* 2007). Many new mechanisms have been created to strengthen research-to-action processes, for example, theory testing and KT effectiveness research, innovations in research synthesis and communication. These mechanisms include the systematic review agencies such as the Cochrane Collaboration, Campbell Collaboration and the UK's National Institute for Health and Clinical Excellence. In addition, policy-oriented research-to-action funding opportunities have been designed to foster collaboration among researchers, policymakers and practitioners, for example CIHR and National Institute for Health (NIH). Considerable KT theory and practice has emerged recently on determinants of research uptake (Nieva *et al.* 2005; LaBresh 2006; Grimshaw 2007; Kitson *et al.* 2008). These are important opportunities for moving research to action in chronic illness.

Stroke as a KT case example

Why use stroke as a case example in this chapter? One could argue that taking a disease-specific approach in a final chapter about the future of chronic illness is in conflict with current chronic illness approaches. However, the intent is not to promote a disease-specific model. The authors use stroke examples as a discrete, real-life chronic illness lens through which the KT challenges that impact chronic illness can be viewed.

Population pyramid changes and increased survival rates mean that stroke incidence is expected to rise at unprecedented rates over the next 25 years (Hallstrom *et al.* 2008). Stroke is a debilitating and life-threatening vascular disease that affects millions of people worldwide each year (Truelsen *et al.* 2001). Sixteen thousand Canadians die from strokes every year (HSF 2006) and stroke survivors often are left with long-term physical and/or mental disability. Family members often experience a heavy caregiver burden (Burvill *et al.* 1995; AHA 2006; HSF 2006).

Stroke, like most chronic illnesses, is a complex condition requiring attention across the full continuum of service from prevention to acute stroke management to community integration. However, care for individuals with most multiple chronic health problems including stroke is often fragmented and less than optimal (Clarfield *et al.* 2001). Both primary and secondary prevention are very poor in many countries and communities despite evidence of effective clinical and population health interventions (Hackam & Spence 2007). Stroke provides a venue for examining the social determinants of health and other contextual factors central to preventing and treating any chronic illness.

The future of chronic illness will be dependent on how knowledge is understood and used within and across the four health pillars: basic, clinical, services and policy and population health. What type of evidence are we talking about? For basic scientists studying stroke, KT strategies concentrate on translational mechanisms from bench to bedside and back again (e.g. animal models of stroke/brain recovery focusing on physical movement and brain protective mechanisms). Clinical stroke research typically focuses on improving current treatment (e.g. thrombolysis, treatment of TIA) and rehabilitation practices and ways to improve patient adherence to prevent stroke or stroke recurrence. In health services and policy, integrated care and stroke units provide a structure within which to integrate evidence. Stroke audits are being increasingly used to examine health policy, outcome and health service delivery. These audits have been extremely influential in convincing policymakers to invest in stroke (DH/Vascular Program 2007a). Population and public health include the generation of data on stroke prevalence, health disparities, social and environmental determinants, health economics and population-based intervention (Lyons & Warner 2005; Feigin & Howard 2008). Similar developments are occurring at an increasing rate across the spectrum of chronic illness, especially where there are funding mechanisms to support KT.

Embedding KT within research agencies and grants

The future of chronic illness will depend, in great measure, on government leadership and investment in KT in the context of research and policy. Substantive transformations have already been made in many countries in the way research is conceptualised and funded in order to foster research use. Funding agencies have begun to provide new opportunities to develop research-to-action KT pipelines that can reduce the gap between researchers and users in health systems, settings such as schools, workplaces, communities, private sector research and development. Funding opportunities have been made available to teams and research centres have been established with KT as a primary function.

In Canada, agencies such as the Networks of Centres of Excellence, CIHR, Public Health Agency of Canada, Canadian Health Services Research Foundation and Social Sciences and Humanities Research Council of Canada have created infrastructure and funding opportunities to support national and international leadership in KT theory and practice. (See Kitson & Bisby 2008 for a review of granting agency developments in KT.) Other KT infrastructure has developed including a new journal, *Implementation Science*, and an increasing amount of KT publications in existing journals.

The National Institute for Health Research in Britain has undergone a substantial transformation, establishing strategic research directions for many elements of chronic illness that include trans-disciplinary collaboration and KT. The UK National Institute for Health and Clinical Excellence (www.nice.org.uk) is a good example of building infrastructure to advance evidence assessment for improved policy and practice. An office of implementation is focused on strategies for uptake of research syntheses and guidelines.

A partnership between researchers and the voluntary sector has advanced research into action on stroke through the Canadian Stroke Strategy. The Canadian Stroke Network (CSN), a national centre of excellence, has been a major contributor in developing research and KT towards improved policy and care. Its partnership with the Heart and Stroke Foundation (HSF) of Canada has fostered policy and practice improvements in every region of Canada. Two characteristics create major challenges for Canada: (a) geography and (b) health service, which is a provincial responsibility with substantially different health resources and commitments to chronic illness in each province.

Each country has its unique contexts including governance and resources (Sabatier 2007). Nevertheless, there are important lessons to be shared among regions and countries as they develop strategies for health improvement and health systems reform. In the stroke world, there is considerable attention to clinical practice in stroke, but relatively little attention is paid to sharing best practice in KT and health systems reform. This situation is changing. The Canadian Stroke Strategy was used as a model for the European Stroke Network. It is expected that the newly established European Stroke Network (funding announced at the European Stroke Conference in Nice, May 2008) will develop as a major force in the uptake of stroke research and evidence and that middle and low resource countries within the European Union will benefit from this collective effort.

Web-based KT innovations

Novel Internet-based approaches have been developed to foster knowledge diffusion and uptake, for example, international theme-related KT networks (The Canadian Dementia Knowledge Translation Network), expert interactive decision tools, modelling processes and access to files and data. KT tools have also been designed to assess KT potential and facilitate access to evidence. For example, in the stroke field, a computer-based assessment tool was designed for examining the KT potential of stroke research (Landry *et al.* 2006). This tool has been adapted for use in other areas such as prevention of oral disease and public health water quality. Another innovative tool is the best practice database such as StrokeEngine, a web-based resource on stroke rehabilitation for health-care providers derived from systematic reviews. The idea is to put evidence into the hands of potential users with a mechanism that can evolve with the generation of new knowledge about stroke rehabilitation (www.canadianstrokenetwork.ca).

In summary, the future of chronic illness will be dependent, in great measure, on how we can mobilise research through KT. Although the early conceptualisations of KT suggested an important but rather simple process, researchers, granting agencies, government health departments and health practitioners have been developing and testing KT processes and infrastructure that support research into action. There are many learnings and innovations that have emerged. However, KT is not without issues. One of these issues is what evidence gets taken up and what does not.

What chronic illness research gets taken up?

The PARiHS framework

Kitson's PARiHS framework is a useful framework for considering the future of chronic illness from a KT perspective. The PARiHS identifies three factors that influence evidence use: the quality of the evidence, the context and the facilitation processes that support research use. Successful implementation (SI) is presented as a function (f) of the nature and type of evidence, the qualities of the context (C) in which the evidence (E) is being introduced and the way the process is being facilitated (F); $SI = f(E,C,F)$. Kitson suggests that the framework can be used as both a diagnostic and an action tool. A number of papers explicate the framework in detail (Kitson *et al.* 1998, 2008).

The PARiHS framework was developed to consider KT in health services but it is also useful in analysing conditions related to the future of health more generally, that is beyond traditional health services such as the social determinants of health. The same three factors (evidence, context and facilitation) are as relevant to evidence use in health-reducing disparities, for instance, or environment and health, as they are in health systems. The framework can account for iterative KT processes and the interaction of the three components. As we have stated earlier, there are challenges in translation and uptake for most types of evidence. A typical KT 'pipeline' (the route from research to action) suggests that there has to be a clear and specific line of research towards technological and policy development (Rogers 1995) and then use. Although rigid, narrow and straight, KT pipelines simply do not exist in the reality of any diffusion process; similar to industrial research and development, they are usually absent in chronic illness.

Chronic illness research and researchers have not usually been organised or mobilised towards development of pipelines or research utilisation (although this is beginning to change). Even when the research has been directed towards change, the policy recommendations are often multi-level changes (poverty reduction; stroke units), highly politically charged and costly.

Some processes, however, are simpler than others. For instance, advances in acute stroke research indicate that early access to emergency services for patients experiencing a stroke is extremely important in order to offer thrombolytic therapy. Approximately 80% of strokes are consequent to a shortage of blood flow to vital areas of the brain, due to an arterial blockage. Thrombolytic therapy offers the opportunity to reopen blocked arteries before permanent damage has occurred. However, thrombolytic drugs are only efficacious when given in the early hours following stroke and can be dangerous, even deadly, if administered to unsuitable patients. The guidelines for seeking emergency attention are straightforward (Hacke *et al.* 2004).

KT in this circumstance is a simpler pathway than the implementation of stroke secondary prevention (e.g. including hypertension control) where compliance typically involves pharmacological adherence and lifestyle modifications. Rates for adherence to both medication and lifestyle recommendations are incredibly poor. Although the evidence of the problem is clear, apart from the benefits of pharmaceuticals and lifestyle modification (Hackam & Spence 2007) there are few clinical or population-level health interventions that have demonstrated efficacious interventions or policy for adherence. The same holds true for implementation of specialised stroke units or integrated care. Although the research indicates that both units and integration result in improved stroke outcome, the exact elements that result in improvement are not clear (Govan *et al.* 2007; Seenan *et al.* 2007).

KT research and the PARiHS framework suggest a set of factors that contribute to research evidence uptake. For example, uptake of evidence or innovation occurs when there is a simple problem with an obvious solution and a clearly identified user whose role it is to address the issue. Also, uptake occurs in instances where the evidence is strong, there is respected leadership and advocacy for uptake, the change requires few resources or does not result in redistribution of resources and there are few political ramifications. Most evidence does not fit these criteria. From a user perspective, Rogers (1995) has argued that the adoption of new ideas/evidence is based on perceived advantage or value-addition of the innovation.

Although there has been no broad-based comparative analysis of what specific health content themes get taken up, many researchers wonder why some chronic illness research with good evidence for action, such as prevention or population health, seems to be sidestepped in current research to policy initiatives. For example, research on social determinants of health such as child development and poverty do not see action compared with pharmaceuticals or clinical practices.

Future attention to chronic illness should provide the impetus to address the lack of a policy interface between health outcomes and social development outcomes. From a health economics perspective, the perceived value of a social-determinants-of-health approach is if it 'unburdens' the health-care system. The other outcomes such as social progress, civil society, social justice, environmental sustainability, human dignity, etc. are not valued as outcomes and any health outcome (such as well-being, sense of belonging) that is broader than a reduced future burden of disease is discounted.

There are many examples of inaction or slow uptake of evidence in prevention, health systems and health determinants (e.g. hypertension; poor workplace air quality; excessive noise). As Lewis commented, we have been mostly a world of disjointed research and pilot projects where good ideas get lost when the research or demonstration money ends. There is often considerable fickleness towards theme areas by politicians. Thus, within government agencies the policy 'product line' changes with incoming bureaucrats or politicians. From both, a research and practice perspective, this continuous shift in focus is deadly (Begin 2007).

Despite the challenges described above, there have been many success stories in addressing chronic illness. We need to learn from these successes. Increasing longevity, for instance, has been attributed to advances in understanding and addressing the determinants of health such as housing, water, etc. Public health advances have resulted in the reduction of infectious disease (perhaps dying of a chronic illness could be considered an advancement from child death due to typhoid fever) and improved care resulting in decreased disability. Policies related to prevention (seat belts, anti-smoking, bike helmets, clear air policies) have resulted in decreased illness and injury. Quality evidence, the case being made and positioned, the focus and strategy then supported by government policy and investment usually lead to engagement by the public and professionals. The UK government has very recently announced its intention to provide leadership on addressing the obesity epidemic with a broad call to public action with commitments of financial support. The documents developed to make the case for setting obesity as a government priority are written to explicate the evidence, to highlight the salience of the issue in contributing to chronic illness and to identify a range of strategies to tackle it (www.dh.gov.uk/en/index.htm, July 23, 2008).

Fixing the context for researchers

Although, Kitson does not explicitly point to the role of researchers in generating and packaging quality evidence in the PARiHS model, the future of chronic illness compels these authors to comment on the research enterprise. What is the context within which researchers are working and how might it be improved to support KT within chronic illness? Where are the goals and the stick-to-it-ness of researchers in seeing applied research made more useable? Are chronic illness researchers working for the same (any common, any specific) goals? What are these? Some might suggest that there would never have been a man on the moon had it been left to health researchers to tackle a moon landing, that is to take on a major task together and carry it through.

Beyond clinical guidelines (and these are often very difficult to apply in most contexts), the work often is not packaged for action. Research production is fragmented and the output is growing exponentially. The required linkages in prevention research, for instance, from population (health and determinants) to health promotion (effective action) to public health (infrastructure and policy), are not usually made. Social scientists who study chronic illness are very adept at identifying problems, not so good at identifying determinants and very poor at predicting optimal policies to address problems. The development of acceptable research methods for complex interventions is a major stumbling block for many chronic illness research questions (Keon 2008).

Carlisle and McMillan (2006) have suggested that innovation is often at the intersection between specialist domains – at points where fields and themes intersect. These points are often the same places where translation occurs. Stepping out of their traditional areas, researchers are now linking up with those from other areas over common, trans-disciplinary problems and approaches. How do we foster such collaborations across disciplines and between research producers and users? Universities are struggling with this concept. Beyond examining new reward systems for such endeavours, there need to be discussions about improving the quality of evidence and KT in the institutions that produce it. There must also be greater attention paid to the role of researchers in applying evidence more efficaciously to chronic illness and positioning the chronic illness debate within challenging and, often-times, illness-producing political contexts.

Researcher hegemony (i.e. consent for the existing power base because it provides research jobs and money) can act as a significant barrier. Money for research is frequently awarded by the same institutional sources that must be lobbied for improvements to health systems. In addition, all research must be critiqued, challenged and reproduced, and is usually insufficient to be definitive. Time is never of the essence when it comes to producing high-quality research. Dissemination is the same – new ideas challenged, debated and often defeated without outside vetting. Another type of hegemony is that it is typically considered unbecoming for a researcher to advocate for one's work/problem to be taken up – that is, the tension between research 'purity' and the pragmatism of research into use (Lyons & McIntyre 2007).

In essence, researchers are small business people trying to stay in business. Every major researcher is first a research manager, working to keep his/her operation solvent, its employees paid and stimulated. Outside suppliers (universities, contractors) have demands that are often not in line with either clinical or population health improvement. Whose demands is a researcher going to meet, particularly when there is usually no client for the results? Impact is measured by grants and scientific publications. KT pipelines that would lead to sustained change are too messy, complicated and beyond a researcher's control. The competition is fierce – with one group critiquing the value of the other. Divide the troops and create rifts. Take my programme – my solution (Lyons & McIntyre 2007).

Collaboration requires communal engagement and shared resources. A recent study by Albert *et al.* (2008) on basic scientists' perceptions of social science in health indicated that up to half of the physical scientists surveyed did not understand or respect the work of social scientists and were not particularly keen to share health research resources with them. Nevertheless, trans-disciplinary research and KT are occurring with funding mechanisms that direct dollars to support such ventures and there are successful examples emerging (Lyons *et al.* 2005). Collaborative ventures like these are new territory for most people (and most countries) and they need to be part of university research training and academic recognition. Future research training must provide opportunities for trainees to work directly with funded trans-disciplinary research teams and across translational boundaries (e.g. bench to bedside to community to policy).

Thus, the future of chronic illness, from a KT perspective, will require thoughtful conceptualisation. What are the key elements in knowledge use? How can they be supported? How can outcomes be measured? How do we set goals and priorities that do not sidestep root causes? How can the research enterprise function more effectively for KT?

Now that the reader is mindful not only of the magnitude of effort required for chronic illness strategies to make a meaningful impact on the problem and the importance of using what we know how to do, the second half of this chapter will specifically apply a KT framework and various components that need to be considered in developing a high-dose solution, using stroke as an example.

Note: Although we have focused on research culture as a factor in KT and chronic illness, we could have just as easily written a section on the working life of public health and health-care practitioners and administrators. However, some of the health system contextual issues that impede knowledge use are discussed in the section on building research use capacity later in the chapter.

Macroscopics: KT and the PARiHS framework

We apply the PARiHS framework in an unusual way. In order to reinforce the theme of substantive change required to address the future of chronic illness, the authors take a *macroscopic and systems* view. Individual pieces of evidence that translate into improved practice are vitally important. However, KT can be advanced through a whole systems perspective – the building of government initiatives that create a supportive culture for KT, innovation and change.

Broad cultural shifts wherein governments are taking chronic illness leadership will ultimately influence the future of chronic illness more than anything. An example is policy leadership in smoking cessation. Other examples include chronic disease and illness strategies, illness-specific strategies such as for cancer, diabetes, etc., approaches to the reduction of health disparities and building and transportation policies related to the built environment and opportunities for physical activity (Hess *et al.* 2008; Sabik & Lie 2008). Many countries and global efforts to improve the quality of care and prevention provide valuable natural experiments in converting research into practice culture. The most promising of these efforts (from a research-to-action perspective) links government action on chronic illness with specific investments in knowledge generation and translation.

Typically, this sort of leadership does not develop in isolation. Clinicians and health professionals are key players. Movers and shakers within voluntary associations, including individuals with health problems and family caregivers, are also extremely important in both lobbying and collaboration. Such tools as national audits which assess the current quality of service, for example Sentinel Stroke Audit in the UK (Clinical Effectiveness and Evaluation Unit, Royal College of Physicians 2007), are very influential. They are often carried out in conjunction with researchers in universities. Celebrities, together with individual and corporate donors, often play major roles in fostering policy agendas for chronic illness.

Government leadership can play a substantive role in enmeshing knowledge use in the roll-out of large chronic illness strategies. These strategies can vary in their scope and function. However, our macroscopic view holds that collective contributions of evidence should move countries to invest substantial resources on improvements in chronic illness prevention and management. In the end, a policy environment that uses evidence in the design of major chronic illness initiatives and a government that uses these initiatives to foster KT are absolutely critical to providing a foundation for reducing the gap between knowledge and action.

Such government leadership enacted through policy investments in carefully crafted health strategies plays a major role in advancing all three of Kitson's KT elements (evidence, context and facilitation) at macro, meso and micro levels within society. In other words, a rising tide lifts all boats. Evidence is enhanced and relevant. The context (research use capacity) is improved. And facilitation occurs as a logical component of the strategy. Communities of practice (or knowledge networks) share problems and approaches so that each site is not reinventing the wheel. Selecting the appropriate level for action is important. For instance, European Union-supported stroke networks and research programmes (e.g. development of standards of care, cross-country comparison of services and health outcomes and conferences) are a lifting mechanism to improve prevention and treatment, particularly in middle- and low-income EU countries.

Before embarking further on the dialogue about optimising government investments in chronic illness, we need to step back and examine the emerging linkages between knowledge creation and its link to chronic illness policy.

Policy containers and the future of chronic illness

Large systemic chronic illness change needs a focus and it needs investment. The term *policy container* is our term to connote the need for a receptacle that will accommodate emergent evidence in chronic illness. The major catalyst for driving integrated care and other major models of chronic illness, is policy, major government positions backed by investment (Kandig 2007). Policy defines, in many cases, the cultural predisposition to addressing chronic illness. It is a critical component in improved health-care and chronic illness outcome – the guide to decisions about allocation of resources. In other words, policy is a key indicator of commitment to health and illness outcomes (Kandig 2007; Matchar *et al.* 2007).

Policy has been conceptualised as the legislative output of the work of elected officials (policymakers) (Sabatier 2007) but a much wider range of health-related decisions and decision makers impact chronic illnesses. Health policy research includes population and outcome studies that contribute to optimising investments to prevent chronic illness and reduce its devastating effects. It includes research on codified decisions made in many governmental and non-governmental settings and at different geographic levels and for different determinant categories. Policy is multifaceted including mission statements, financing, strategies, organisational structures, services (including access) and organisational capacity to use evidence.

Chronic illness researchers and practitioners have begun to pay attention to policy as they understand more fully how it becomes the link between research and practice and influences the development of a whole system's culture oriented to the use of evidence. What sorts of policies positively impact chronic illness? What might the future hold if we were able, with the help of evidence, to build strong policy investments in chronic illness prevention and treatment?

Reich *et al.* (2008) suggest that if we are serious about a bright future for health and improved health outcomes, we require systems approaches, especially in tackling global health problems. They state that systems are needed to generate solutions, incentives and competence. A health system is a complex socio-economic structure that provides both prevention and curative services for people. When a health system works well, it produces good results, for example, Japan's record on health outcomes.

A health system supports specific activities in much the same way that a computer's basic hardware and software support the ability to run specific programs.

(Reich et al. 2008)

Likewise, translation of knowledge into action for chronic illness needs central government and health systems to provide the basic foundation and infrastructure if we are to realise a future that supports individual and group KT successes in prevention and treatment.

Whole systems thinking for organisational change must include approaches to improve service, measures to assess capacity to use evidence and analysis of the barriers to implementation of evidence. Several researchers are using systems, or whole systems approaches, to build an infrastructure to support KT. For example, Wolfe *et al.* (2007) are working on the development of a European Implementation Score (EIS) for KT using vascular health (stroke) as a case example. Comparing European countries on the EIS could provide one of the first major analyses of uptake and its determinants.

The advantage of a large government strategy on chronic illness or on specific conditions such as stroke means that there is a receptor and container for new knowledge as it emerges. Through knowledge networks, brokers, forums and audits to examine progress in research use, processes are put in place for knowledge use and more equitable use, both within and across countries.

The future of chronic illness: systems change using stroke examples

The following are seven examples of how emerging evidence in stroke can be applied to prevent and manage illness and how bold leadership can create a culture for chronic illness research use. The seven examples include (a) integrated care frameworks, (b) stroke strategies, (c) international collaboration, (d) access to service, (e) public engagement, (f) predictive modelling and (g) research use capacity.

Stroke and integrated care frameworks

Integrated care has become a common framework and a strategic policy container for chronic illness evidence and best practice (Plochg & Klazinga 2002). From a KT perspective, the thinking is that organised systems of prevention and care around an implementation strategy provide the foundation for health system financial investments, human resource coordination and development and the mechanism for effective uptake of evidence through practice guidelines, training and research.

Elements of service in stroke policy frameworks, for instance, are typically portrayed as prevention, acute care, rehabilitation and community service nested within a coordinated system and overarching supportive health and social policies, for example geriatrics and cardiovascular disease, chronic disease prevention and management, health disparities and systems of payment. One of the most recent strategies, the National Stroke Strategy in England, contained a very detailed analysis of service components for chronic illness with a strong self-management perspective. Countries such as Canada, Scotland and Australia have also initiated evidence-based integrated care for stroke (DH 2000; Woods 2001; National Health Service for Scotland 2005). This approach has also been used for other conditions such as diabetes and stroke and by some countries such as Wales for chronic illness, more generally. The precise outcomes of complex health systems change, such as integrated care, are methodologically challenging; however, studies of integrated care have shown improvements in quality of care, patient outcomes and clinical expertise (Audit Scotland 2005; Minkman *et al.* 2005; Canadian Stroke Network 2006).

Deciding among competing chronic illness models is a challenge: integrated care; disease-specific, social determinants; health outcome versus quality of life. The proponents of these models end up competing with each other because of scarce resources, multiple outcome orientations and population health needs, and hence the focus is lost. In the development of government chronic illness strategies there are normally hundreds of actors (researchers, advocacy associations, lawyers and politicians), each with potentially different interests, values and preferences (Sabatier 2007). Similar to the movement for climate change, scientists across disciplines must come together with a united voice, pool skills and research and provide a sense of clarity for policymakers to take action on leading issues. An example of such an issue is the current epidemic of youth obesity.

181

National stroke strategies

Chronic illness policy strategies such as the Ontario Stroke Strategy (Canada) or the National Health Stroke Strategy in England are important natural (intervention) experiments to examine the effectiveness of approaches that use knowledge in improving the quality of prevention and treatment. These strategies include a plan of action for improving stroke care, financial commitments, and most importantly, the designation of stroke as a priority and focus for assessment. The following are potential roles of stroke and other chronic illness strategies in moving research into action:

1. To apply evidence in key decisions about where and how to invest, including establishing stroke (or chronic illness) as a priority
2. To examine process and outcomes of interventions in diverse environments (what works, in what situations, for whom) (Pawson 2006)
3. To train health professionals in evidence use
4. To facilitate and support the use of evidence, for example, create networks and other structures that support research adoption and adaptation for specific setting; sharing best practice and its use in annual forums and the Internet
5. To create requests for research application (joined-up with research granting agencies) on important but under-researched areas central to addressing prevention and management
6. To fund well-constructed health service and population health demonstration projects
7. To examine how evidence gets contextualised for different geographic, ethnic and other conditions

Lists like the one given above could be formed into a KT lens that could be applied to the design and implementation of chronic illness strategies of the future. This approach would ensure that we are optimising the knowledge development and use opportunities that then could be shared within and across national boundaries.

How can evidence be applied strategically during the formation of a chronic illness strategy? Some research has shown that different types of evidence are required at each stage in the development and implementation of large-scale strategies for the prevention and treatment of chronic illness. The role of evidence was examined in the development of the Ontario Stroke System (a $30 million per year health policy initiative to improve stroke care in Ontario, Canada). Researchers identified key stages in the implementation process and the various types of evidence mobilised at each stage (Cameron *et al.* 2007).

Researchers working together across disciplines can play critical roles in the synthesis and communication of chronic illness research. Researchers in population health (health and determinants), public health (prevention infrastructure) and health promotion (strategy/action), together with clinician-scientists, can paint a clearer picture of what needs to be done and what might be the best approaches, together with providing economic data regarding cost benefit. This work, which mobilises many sorts of knowledge, must be a collaborative venture among researchers, practitioners and advocacy associations with commitment over time if change is to occur. There is a clear link between research and advocacy here.

Fostering international collaboration

As has been discussed earlier, chronic illness is a global health issue for both low- and middle-income countries. Efforts to tackle this issue on an international basis need to be supported. Strategies for addressing chronic illness have been developed across countries and regions, such as through Pan American Health Organization (PAHO), World Health Organization (WHO), etc. CARMEN, the acronym for the Spanish Conjuncto de Acciones para la Reducion Multifactorial de Enfermedades No Transmisibles, is an initiative of PAHO/WHO to promote the prevention of non-communicable diseases throughout the Americas. CARMEN includes 22 countries and 9 collaborating groups. The aims are to promote evidence-based practice, to share strategies and develop demonstration sites for interventions in prevention and control of chronic illness. For instance, one project involves mobilisation for cardiovascular health promotion through lay personnel in Chile, Guatemala and Argentina. The work is framed within a chronic care model including five main components: delivery system design, decision support, self-management support, clinical information systems and community services (CARMEN/PAHO 2008).

How does the international approach apply to improvements in the prevention and management of stroke? The Helsingborg Declaration 2006 on European Stroke Strategies (Kjellstrom *et al.* 2007) is one example of the potential lifting mechanism of international collaboration to enhance stroke health policy and practice in the European Union. The Declaration states that by 2015 all persons in Europe with stroke should have access to a continuum of care in the acute phase including rehabilitation and secondary prevention. Clear goals for improving outcomes, the means to achieve them and evaluation, are outlined. The document also calls for a system to be established to incorporate new research into stroke care. These statements pool efforts of governments, researchers and clinicians to improve conditions, and avoid duplication and fragmentation of resources and efforts.

Access to service

We normally think of access to health service in terms of who gets service and the quality of service provision. Access can also be conceived of as where we invest, as prioritisation based on factors such as social determinants of health. KT can be very valuable in examining cultural variations in access to and use of services. Advances have been made in identifying the etiology of chronic illness and determinants of chronic illness burden and outcome. New methods have been developed to examine the etiology of chronic illness. In the area of stroke, 'stroke belt' research (geographic areas of high incidence and mortality) and other determinants studies examine regional, socio-economic and ethno-cultural variations in stroke prevalence and outcome. Stroke belt analyses and other population health approaches to the epidemiology of chronic illness contribute to identifying risk factors for chronic illness and increase clarity about where policy should be directed. Interestingly, the stroke belt work suggests that early life exposures (e.g. where one lives as a child) are important in explaining stroke mortality (El-Saed & Kuller 2007; Glymour *et al.* 2007). What do these data suggest for research and KT on stroke and other health problems? What are these early life exposures? What are the implications for stroke prevention strategies?

Are those who need care getting it, especially those in low socio-economic groups? A WHO study found that 87% of the 5.7 million people who die annually from stroke live in low- or middle-income countries. These people are often unable to access stroke units or new drugs. Primary prevention and adequate stroke treatment are essential (Strong *et al.* 2007). A related study on urbanisation and poverty levels suggests a relation between inner city slums and strokes (Herng-Ching *et al.* 2007). Following a study to quantify the socio-economic gap in long-term health outcomes after stroke and related health-care utilisation, it was concluded that greater clarity is needed in policy decisions about access, for example, coordinated care investments and disadvantaged groups (van den Bos *et al.* 2002).

High-quality acute care is an important element in chronic illness treatment and the reduction of disability. Efforts have increased recently in the documentation of the quality of care as a major factor in determining policy investments and in the use of evidence in improving care. Stroke units, for example, contribute to a reduction in deaths, dependency, the need for institutional care (Dennis & Langhorne 1994; SUTC 1997) and hospital stays (Jorgensen *et al.* 1995; Wentworth & Atkinson 1996). Stroke units have been shown to be less expensive than traditional ward care (SUTC 1997) and result in higher patient satisfaction (Mayor 2005). Surveys of patient satisfaction show that having a service system that is accessible and helps to coordinate care is associated with a significantly more positive patient and caregiver experience (Schoen *et al.* 2007). However, these types of stroke units are not present in most regions of the world.

A study of stroke units in 886 hospitals in 25 European countries provided valuable insights into the current status of acute care for stroke. Less than 10% of hospitals had optimal facilities and in 40% the minimal level of service was not available (Leys *et al.* 2007). Access to stroke care units in public hospitals in Australia was compared with 1999 levels. Findings showed that although progress had been made, the percentage of people accessing stroke units was approximately 20% as compared with 70% in Sweden. Policy to improve access to stroke units was recommended (Cadilhac *et al.* 2006). Comparisons of leading and lagging countries, regions or health-care facilities may be seen as victimisation of low resource or specially challenged environments. However, they have proven quite effective in drawing attention to disparities in service quality and increased investment in finding resources and approaches to challenged environments. In the future, inadequate access service defined by evidence will likely become a growing legal issue.

Although there have been major advances in acute care for stroke in the Province of Ontario, Canada, deficiencies were reported in post-stroke services such as depression (Saposnik & Kapral 2007). Correspondingly, a rehabilitation consensus conference was held in Canada to identify priority areas for programmes and research. Areas in need of research and action included multi-modal programmes for reintegration, rehabilitation for severe stroke, cognitive rehabilitation and research on the timing and intensity for two areas: aphasia therapy and therapy after mild to moderate stroke events (Bayley *et al.* 2007). In another study, post-hospital care was the theme of an analysis of seven hospitals in Taipei (Chuang *et al.* 2007). These authors argued that the ageing society must establish improved stroke service as a health-care priority. The value in having KT infrastructure is that these studies of access to quality care do not sit on a shelf, but are considered for action as a function of mechanisms such as practice guidelines (and their implementation), stroke strategies and stroke knowledge networks.

Public engagement in knowledge use and policy

A promising approach to moving research to action via countrywide strategies is the development of evidence-based plans brought together with new styles of public engagement. For instance, the National Health Service in England developed a comprehensive consultation document on stroke to stimulate debate on how best to prevent and treat stroke (DH/Vascular Program/Stroke Team 2007b). This document includes considerable detail about the components of integrated care (including prevention) written in language that is understandable by policymakers and the public. The document provides useful frameworks that outline elements of care including post-stroke care (p. 34), discussion questions and stories that accompany the draft recommendations. This approach can be applied to other specific conditions, and to chronic illness more generally, as an example of how to engage the public in dialogue about making chronic illness a central policy issue and the key components that need to be included. These exercises must be used in the allocation of resources, not merely held as political events with the appearance of agency and inclusion. At the local level, health professionals and citizens must be engaged in local improvements to health and health care. A sense of ownership, pride and accountability will build high-quality community health and a healthy community.

The promise of predictive modelling in chronic illness policy

There are many mechanisms at play in making substantive investments in addressing chronic illness. As we have said earlier, some of the biggest constraints in many countries have been the constantly changing agenda and the reluctance to make major long-term commitments. Indeed, attempts at setting priorities in health service have been extremely challenging, with mixed results (Sabik & Lie 2008). Keeping with the theme of strategic investment in chronic illness prevention and management, we need to be developing and using tools that will help guide decision-making. How do we get the dose–response correct? For instance, what will it take to substantially reduce risk factors for stroke?

Predictive modelling is a developing approach that has considerable potential for marrying chronic illness research with policy. Accurate estimates of the burden of the target problem coupled with the likely outcome of policy options are valuable contributors to policy decision-making (Petticrew *et al.* 2004). Predictive modelling is related to systematic reviews of health research. Systematic reviews are typically developed with a predictive function in mind; that is, what does the evidence suggest about what works, with whom, under what conditions? As chronic illness is complex and variable, predictive modelling must be supplemented with qualitative research.

The role of modelling is not to establish truth, but to guide decision-making (Weinstein *et al.* 2001). Predictive modelling is an approach that is frequently used in business (www.clockwork-solutions.com/) and in physical science to display optimal policy guidance. Quantitative methods include structural modelling and policy simulation (Bronnenberg *et al.* 2005) – optimal decision processes, as well as spatial micro-simulation (physical or geographic presentation of predictive data) (Mitchell *et al.* 2002).

Spatial micro-simulation is a method used to estimate demographic and socio-economic characteristics of individuals and households. Ballas *et al.* (2004) have used this approach to develop a spatial decision support system for the Leeds City Council, UK. The model can be calibrated to provide analyses of 'what is' and probability estimates of 'what if' on a range of possible policy scenarios. Some work has been done with predictive modelling of health-care policy and population health characteristics (Ballas *et al.* 2006), but very little on preventive health policy.

Three recent papers have used predictive modelling related to improvement to stroke policy. In a paper by Whitfield *et al.* (2006), economic predictive modelling was used to demonstrate the 'invest to save' approach in building an economic argument for funding public health prevention to reduce the cardio-vascular disease (CVD) risk. The idea here is that putting money into prevention saves money down the road.

A paper by Matchar *et al.* (2007) described how a multivariate risk prediction equation using the Duke Stroke Model was developed to estimate stroke admissions and their financial impact. The resultant simulation model was used to produce a legislative document reporting on the potential health and economic impact of improved stroke services in Mississippi. From a knowledge exchange perspective, a complex statistical approach was translated into a report written to be understandable at the policy level. Both the predictive model and the reporting mechanisms may be of value to other jurisdictions aiming to identify optimal investments in stroke and/or other chronic illnesses.

Researchers have also used predictive modelling in stroke secondary prevention (Rothwell 2007). For example, Hackam and Spence (2007) used predictive modelling to examine the potential effectiveness of combining multiple interventions in secondary prevention of stroke. It was shown that at least 80% of recurrent cerebrovascular events might be prevented by incorporating five proven clinical strategies: dietary modification, exercise, aspirin, a statin and a hypertensive agent. Additional therapies such as smoking cessation increase effectiveness.

Building research use capacity – linking policy with practice

For national policy to facilitate change there must be a thoughtful linkage to regional and local levels of service. In health systems, KT, the dynamic dance between policy and grass roots activity is extremely important. Recent observations of the implementation of UK stroke strategy demonstrate this dynamic (and tension) – at what level action is taken, how to pool expertise and processes versus reinventing the wheel in every regional and local health system, but, how to engage those on the front lines in determining change.

How can government investments be designed to reduce the tension between policy imperatives and the support of local innovation and development? It is fine to write guidelines, but can they get activated on the ground and in lower resource environments? As Kitson *et al.* (2008) and Dopson and Fitzgerald (2005) have shown, players on the ground need to be intimately involved in the change process and they need resources to support them. Application of evidence is complex, context-related and is about individuals and organisations, often at many levels.

Health systems face the challenge of maintaining existing services, while responding to demands for improving the quality of patient care, accountability and cost-effectiveness. Research evidence that suggests changes to policy and practice creates added stress because it must be incorporated within existing structures. Researchers have called for new theoretical approaches to aid in understanding research uptake and informing action-oriented efforts to enhance capacity for research use (Grimshaw *et al.* 2004; Eccles *et al.* 2005).

Quality improvement in care based on a policy agenda requires changes in individual and group behaviours. Clarifying barriers and facilitators to change are key elements of this process, although some conditions are context specific (Robinson *et al.* 2007). An example of how research can inform evidence use is a mixed methods approach to examine readiness for quality improvement from the perspectives of staff, patients and administrators in acute care.

The following factors were found to influence the climate of change: the nature of past efforts to use evidence in organisational change, working environment, team climate and organisational stability (Hamilton *et al.* 2007). These data were then used to inform the development of an implementation strategy. This approach may be of value to health systems examining the climate for change and working to improve it.

The capacity for research uptake within health systems can vary substantially as a function of resources (Tugwell *et al.* 2006). Alvaro and her colleagues argue that organisational resources are critical for adaptation and change stemming from evidence-based practice. This argument is supported by a large body of KT literature, which has identified organisational factors affecting research uptake (for a review see Alvaro *et al.* 2007). What are these organisational resources and how do resources function to support or contain research use?

A programme of research applied the Conservation of Resources Theory (Hobfoll 1989, 1998) to knowledge use. The researchers discovered a number of interesting features about organisational resources and how they function:

1. Organisational resources that are important to research use include human resources, organisational culture, economic resources and condition resources. Condition resources include situations and states that open up access to new

resources; for example, a national strategy on stroke that includes new funding to support system change.

2. Change carries with it the threat of resource loss. When threatened by potential resource loss resulting from evidence-informed change, health systems personnel tend to guard resources and resist change.

3. Research use depends upon the presence of an organisational culture that maintains some flexibility in how its resources are distributed and used. In other words, research use depends on resource optimisation. Resource manipulation, mobilisation and substitution contribute to the elasticity (and resiliency) necessary for making the changes to health systems based on research evidence (Alvaro *et al.* 2007).

Kitson's PARiHS framework speaks to the important role of facilitation in research use – a mechanism to contextualise evidence and also to enhance resilience and resource optimisation (Kitson *et al.* 2008).

Two promising interventions that have been proposed to help the evolution of an evidence-informed health system are the use of knowledge brokers and the creation of knowledge networks. A knowledge broker is someone who brings people together and builds relationships to facilitate the sharing of ideas and evidence that helps health-care stakeholders provide better care (Canadian Health Services Research Foundation 2003).

Knowledge networks (or communities of practice) are groups of experts (researchers, practitioners, policymakers) working together on addressing a common issue (Contractor & Monge 2002). A study by Lyons *et al.* (2006) was conducted on the use of knowledge brokers and networks for health system improvements in stroke care. Combining the interventions increased effectiveness and sustainability. The research project used the PARiHS framework to understand how contextual and facilitation factors (knowledge brokers and knowledge networks) affected the adoption of evidence related to improving stroke care by four provincial health-care systems in Canada. The knowledge network supported the work of the knowledge broker during the research project and helped to sustain the work after the project was completed. The following themes were important to the success of the intervention:

1. The context – conditions that impacted the province's ability to make health system changes, for example, few financial and human resources for KT, bias against stroke (an older person's condition), time to effect change (length of the project) and health district support for change
2. Qualities of the knowledge broker – relationship builder, champion, personal knowledge of stroke evidence and organisational change, whether the knowledge broker was working inside or outside of the government
3. Qualities of the network – the nature of the partnership between government and advocacy organisation, regional learning and support and knowledge of evidence and implementation
4. Knowledge uptake – diffusion of knowledge, change in knowledge

Results demonstrated that a knowledge broker can successfully facilitate health system change; however, the work needs to be contextualised and sustainable. Other KT-oriented relationships need to be established and maintained. The knowledge network provided a structure for relationships to flourish. The network allowed researchers, practitioners and health-care decision-makers to identify areas of common interest, created linkages outside of the research project to support the work of the knowledge broker during the research project and sustain the work after the research project was completed. A key factor in the success of both interventions was contextualising evidence to the setting.

Evidence-based practice guidelines often go unused. Examples of *practical* methods for health system quality improvement are essential to policymakers, administrators and clinicians. A framework and collaborative process was developed by LaBresh (2006) for diagnosing barriers to acute stroke care system redesign. This initiative resulted in the several tools (e.g. GWTG-Stroke) to support system change.

Research use capacity is not only an artifact of the working environment but also a function of training. Craig and Smith (2007) used stroke as a case example to illustrate the importance of linking health-care policy to education policy. Academic and medical training must include methods for translation of research into clinical delivery. This statement could also be made for policymakers and community-based service providers. Unfortunately, many project grants are too small or of too short a duration to include a proper best practice review and quality evaluation. Also, knowledge of the broader policy context should be part of clinical training across disciplines.

KT-friendly policy must include appropriate funds dedicated to health-care systems re-modelling. Change requires resources (Alvaro *et al.* 2007). Using the PARiHS framework, these authors have argued that broad strategies/policies are needed that provide the 'lifting mechanisms' to support research into action related to high-quality research and evaluation. Secondly, resources are central to a health system's capacity to adapt (contextualise) and use evidence; and thirdly, there needs to be interface among macro, meso and micro levels within a health system to coordinate and support research use. The policy process should contain opportunities for both bottom-up and top-down activities and these activities need to be somewhat in synchrony.

Conclusion

The authors of this chapter have provided an overview of the growing problem of chronic illness and the challenges in trying to address it. We took a small bite out of this enormous subject by zeroing in on KT. We introduced the concept, provided examples of advances and the new directions being taken to move research to action and raised questions about why some research gets taken up and some does not. The role of the research enterprise in supporting this process is extremely important to consider. Macroscopic systems strategies were examined in order to build a foundation that could eventually transform the fundamentals of prevention and care. Individual pieces of evidence that translate into improved practice are vitally important. However, KT can be advanced through a whole systems perspective including the broad contributions of evidence that move countries to invest substantial focus and resources towards improvements in chronic illness prevention and management.

The examples from stroke were given to demonstrate the breadth of research questions and approaches being used to understand and act on chronic illnesses. This work has yielded policy-relevant outcomes. It also resulted in outputs such as new research approaches related to strategies and elements of care, optimising policy investments and KT.

There is growing recognition that the actions of past generations have set the stage for major challenges for future generations in environment, poverty and health. Excesses such as fossil fuel overuse, decisions that have often favoured economics over health and social and environmental determinants of health are forcing us to attend to chronic illness as never before. In addition, advances in public health and illness treatment have contributed to the growing burden of chronic illness. There is need for population evidence combined with evidence of effectiveness, together with policy research, together with clinical research on approaches with individuals and groups. This is the future of prevention and management of chronic illness.

Despite the data on chronic illness mortality and morbidity that compel poli-cymakers to act, clarity about effective solutions and policymaker roles in these solutions is needed. In particular, how can we focus research and policy on prevention and treatment of underserved people and regions? Given the heavy burden of chronic illness in developing countries, how can evidence be used to make the case that it receives greater attention in global health (Fuster *et al.* 2007)? Lastly, in order to advance the quality of care and improve health outcomes, how can policy include commitments to research as a key component of chronic illness strategies?

The authors provided these ideas in a world where high-quality evidence is but one, albeit central, component in helping to make the 'right' practice or policy decision (Sabatier 2007), and dealing with the social and economic tensions listed earlier. Scientific evidence, especially in complex systems, needs to be coupled with a culture that supports innovation and change, including incentives, advanced technology, organisational knowledge structures, processes of team decision-making in ethics and health systems and a political culture prepared to take serious and sustained action on chronic illness.

Acknowledgements
Very sincere thanks to Alastair Buchan who hosted Renee Lyons at the John Radcliffe Hospital and Green College during her 2008 sabbatical at the University of Oxford; Tony Hakim and the Canadian Stroke Network for supporting impor-tant research into knowledge translation and stroke; and Roger Boyle, National Director for Heart Disease and Stroke, Department of Health, National Health

Service, UK, for many inspirational meetings about government roles in strategies that move chronic illness research towards improved prevention and treatment. Also, thanks to Sandra Crowell and Meredith Flannery for assistance in the final preparation of the chapter.

References

Abegunde, D.O., Mathers, C., Adam, T., Ortegon, M., Strong, K. (2007) The burden and costs of chronic disease in low-income and middle-income countries. *Lancet* **370**: 1929–1938.

Albert, M., Lamberge, S., Hodges, B.D., Regehr, G., Lingard, L. (2008) Biomedical scientists' perception of the social sciences in health research. *Social Sciences and Medicine* **66**: 2520–2531.

Alvaro, C., Lyons, R., Warner, G. *et al.* (2007) *Conservation of Resources Theory and Knowledge Translation in Health Systems.* Manuscript submitted for publication.

American Diabetes Association. (2006) Nutrition recommendations and interventions for diabetes – 2006. A position statement of the American Diabetes Association. *Diabetes Care* **29**: 2140–2157.

American Heart Association. (2006) Heart Disease and Stroke Statistics – 2006 Update: A report from the American Heart Association Statistics Committee and Stroke Statistics Subcommittee. *Circulation* **113**: e85–e151.

Audit Scotland. (2005) *Overview of the Performance of the NHS in Scotland 2004/ 2005* from www.audit-scotland.gov.uk/publications/pubs2005.htm (accessed in 2008).

Ballas, D., Clarke, G., Dorling, D., Rigby, J., Wheeler, B. (2006) Using geographical information systems and spatial microsimulation for the analysis of health inequalities. *Health Informatics Journal* **12**: 65–79.

Ballas, D., Kingston, R., Stillwell, J., Jin, J. (April 2004) *Building a Spatial Microsimulation Decision Support System.* Paper presented at the Proceedings of the 7th AGILE Conference on Geographic Information Science, Heraklion.

Bayley, M.T., Hurdowar, A., Teasell, R. *et al.* (2007) Priorities for stroke rehabilitation and research: results of a 2003 Canadian stroke network consensus conference. *Archives of Physical Medicine and Rehabilitation* **88**: 526–528.

Begin, M. (2007) Do I see a demand? From "medicare" to health for all. *Journal of Public Sector Management* **37**: 15.

van den Bos, G.A.M., Smits, J.P., Westert, G.P., van Straten, A. (2002) Socioeconomic variations in the course of stroke: unequal health outcomes, equal care? *Journal of Epidemiology and Community Health* **56**: 943–948.

Bringewatt, R.J. (2003) *Check List for Chronic Care Reform.* National Chronic Care Consortium: Washington, DC. Retreived 2 February 2008, from www.ncconline.org/pdf/ChronicCareChecklist.pdf.

Bronnenberg, B.J., Rossi, P., Vilcassim, N.J. (2005) Structural modeling and policy simulation. *Journal of Marketing Research* **42**: 22–26.

Burvill, P., Johnson, G., Jamrozik, K., Anderson, C., Stewart-Wynne, E., Chakera, T. (1995) Prevalence of depression after stroke: the Perth community stroke study. *The British Journal of Psychiatry* **166**: 320–327.

Cadilhac, D.A., Lalor, E.E., Pearce, D.C., Levi, C.R., Donnan, G.A. (2006) Access to stroke care units in Australian public hospitals: facts and temporal progress. *Internal Medicine Journal* **36**: 700–704.

Cameron, J.I., Rappolt, S., Lewis, M., Lyons, R., Warner, G., Silver, F. (2007) Development and implementation of the Ontario stroke system: the use of evidence. *International Journal of Integrated Care* **7**: 1–10.

Canadian Health Services Research Foundation. (2003) *The Theory and Practice of Knowledge Brokering in Canada's Health System*. Canadian Health Services Research Foundation: Ottawa.

Canadian Institutes of Health Research (CIHR). (2008) http://www.cihr-irsc.gc.ca/e/29418.html.

Canadian Stroke Network. (2006) *The Social and Economic Impact of Providing Organized Stroke Care in Canada*. Retrieved 3 January 2007, from www.canadianstrokestrategy.ca/technical_docs/organizedstrokecareoct06.pdf.

Carlisle, Y., McMillan, E. (2006) Innovation in organizations from a complex adaptive systems perspective. *Emergence, Complexity, and Organizations* **8**: 2–9.

CARMEN/PAHO. (2008) CARMEN Network. Retrieved 1 August 2008, from www.paho.org/English/AD/DPC/NC/carmen-info.htm.

Carnes, B.A., Olshansky, S.J. (2007) A realist view of aging, mortality, and future longevity. *Population and Development Review* **33**: 367–381.

Choi, B.C.K., McQueen, D.V., Puska, P. *et al.* (2008) Enhancing global capacity in the surveillance, prevention, and control of chronic diseases: seven themes to build upon. *Journal of Epidemiology and Community Health* **62**: 391–397.

Chronic Disease Prevention Alliance of Canada. (January 2004) *The Cost of Chronic Disease in Canada*. Ottawa.

Chuang, K.Y., Wu, S.C., Dai, Y.T., Ma, A.H.S. (2007) Post-hospital care of stroke patients in Taipei: use of services and policy implications. *Health Policy* **82**: 28–36.

Clarfield, A.M., Bergman, H., Kane, R. (2001) Fragmentation of care for frail older people – an international problem. Experience from three countries: Israel, Canada, and the United States. *Journal of the American Geriatrics Society* **49**: 1714–1721.

Clinical Effectiveness and Evaluation Unit, Royal College of Physicians. (April 2007) *National Sentinel Stroke Audit, 2006*. London.

Contractor, N.S., Monge, P.R. (2002) Managing knowledge networks. *Management Communications Quarterly* **16**: 249–259.

Craig, L.E., Smith, L.N. (2007) The interaction between policy and education using stroke as an example [Electronic Version]. *Nurse Education Today* **28**: 77–84.

Crombie, K., Irvine, L., Elliott, L., Wallace, H. (2005) *Closing the Health Inequalities Gap: An International Perspective*. World Health Organization: Europe.

Davis, D. (2007) *The Secret History of the War on Cancer*. Basic Books: New York.

Dennis, M., Langhorne, P. (1994) Fortnightly review: so stroke units save lives: where do we go from here? *British Medical Journal* **309**: 1273–1277.

Department of Health. (2000) *The NHS Plan: A Summary*. London.

Department of Health. (2004) *Chronic Disease Management: A Compendium of Information*. London.

Department of Health. (2006) *Tackling Health Inequalities: Status Report on the Programme for Action – 2006 Update of Headline Indicators*. London.

Department of Health/Vascular Program. (2007a) *National Stroke Strategy for England*. London.

Department of Health/Vascular Program/Stroke Team. (2007b) *A New Ambition for Stroke: A Consultation on a National Strategy*. London.

Dopson, S., Fitzgerald, L. (2005) *Knowledge to Action*. Oxford University Press: Oxford.

Eccles, M., Grimshaw, J., Walker, A., Johnson, M., Pitts, N. (2005) Response to "the OFF theory of research utilization". *Journal of Clinical Epidemiology* **58**: 117–118.

El-Saed, A., Kuller, L.H. (2007) Is the stroke belt worn from childhood: current knowledge and future directions. *Stroke* **38**: 2403–2404.

Feigin, V.L., Howard, G. (2008) The importance of epidemiological studies should not be downplayed. *Stroke* **39**: 1–2.

Fuster, V., Voute, J., Hunn, M., Smith, S.C. Jr. (2007) Low priority of cardiovascular and chronic diseases on the global health agenda. *Circulation* **116**: 1966–1970.

Gibbons, M. (1999) Science's new social contract with society. *Nature* **402**: C81–C84.

Glymour, M.M., Avendano, M., Berkman, L.F. (2007) Is the 'Stroke Belt' worn from childhood? *Stroke* **38**: 2415–2421.

Govan, L., Langhorne, P., Weir, C. (2007) Does the prevention of complications explain the survival benefit of organized inpatient (stroke unit) care? *Stroke* **38**: 2536–2540.

Graham, I.D., Tetroe, J. (2007) How to translate health research knowledge into effective healthcare action. *Healthcare Quarterly* **10**: 20–22.

Grimshaw, J. (September 2007) *Improving the Scientific Basis of Health Care Research Dissemination and Implementation*. Presentation at NIH Conference on "Building the Science of Dissemination and Implementation in the Service of Public Health", Bethesda, MD.

Grimshaw, J., Eccles, M., Tetroe, J. (2004) Implementing clinical guidelines: current evidence and future implications. *Journal of Continuing Education in the Health Professions* **24**: S31–S37.

Grol, R., Grimshaw, J. (2003) From best evidence to best practice: effective implementation of change in patients' care. *The Lancet* **362**: 1225.

Hackam, D.G., Spence, J.D. (2007) Combining multiple approaches for the secondary prevention of vascular events after stroke: a quantitative modeling study. *Stroke* **38**: 1881–1885.

Hacke, W., Donnan, G., Fieschi, C. *et al.* (2004) Association of outcome with early stroke treatment: pooled analysis of ATLANTIS, ECASS, and NINDS rt-PA stroke trials. *Lancet* **363**: 768–774.

Hallstrom, B., Jonsson, A., Nerbreand, C., Norrving, B., Lindgre, A. (2008) Stroke incidence and survival in the beginning of the 21st century and projections into the future. *Stroke* **39**: 10–15.

Hamilton, S., McLaren, S., Mulhall, A. (2007) Assessing organizational readiness for change: use of diagnostic analysis prior to the implementation of a multidisciplinary assessment for acute stroke care. *Implementation Science* **2**: 21.

Harper, S. (2006) *Ageing Societies*. Hodder Arnold: London.

Heart and Stroke Foundation of Canada. (2006) *General Information – Stroke Statistics*. Retrieved 5 January 2007, from ww2.heartandstroke.ca.

Herng-Ching, L., Yen-Ju, L., Tsai-Ching, L., Chin-Shyan, C., Wen-Ta, C. (2007) Urbanization and stroke prevalence in Taiwan: analysis of a nationwide survey. *Journal of Urban Health: Bulletin of the New York Academy of Medicine* **84**: 604–614.

Hess, C., Schwartz, S., Rosenthal, J., Snyder, A., Weil, A. (2008) *State Health Policies Aimed at Promoting Excellent Systems: A Report on State's Roles in Health Systems Performance*. National Academy for State Health Policy: Washington, DC.

Hobfoll, S.E. (1989) Conservation of resources: a new attempt at conceptualizing stress. *American Psychologist* **44**(3): 513–524.

Hobfoll, S.E. (1998) *Stress, Culture and Community*. Plenum Press: New York.

Jorgensen, H.S., Nakayana, H., Raaschou, H.O., Larsen, K., Hubbe, P., Olsen, T.S. (1995) The effect of a stroke unit: reductions in mortality discharge rate to nursing home, length of hospital stay and cost. *Stroke* **26**: 1178–1182.

Kandig, D. (2007) Understanding population health terminology. *The Milbank Quarterly* **85**: 139–161.

Keon, W.J. (2008) *Population Health Policy: International Perspectives. First Report of the Subcommittee on Population Health of the Standing Senate Committee on Social Affairs, Science, and Technology*. Retrieved 6 November 2007, from www.parl.gc.ca.

Kerner, J.F. (2006) Dullest translation versus knowledge integration: a "funder's" perspective. *The Journal of Continuing Education in the Health Professions* **26**: 72–80.

Kickbusch, I., McCann, W., Sherbon, T. (2008) Adelaide revisited: from healthy public policy to health in all policies. *Health Promotion International* **23**: 1–3.

Kitson, A.L., Bisby, M. (June 2008) *Speeding up the Spread. Putting KT Research into Practice and Developing an Integrated KT Collaborative Research Agenda*. Discussion paper of the KT08 Forum. Alberta Heritage Foundation for Medical Research: Banff.

Kitson, A.L., Harvey, G., McCormack, B. (1998) Enabling the implementation of evidence-based practice: a conceptual framework. *Quality in Health Care* **7**: 149–158.

Kitson, A.L., Rycroft-Malone, J., Harcey, G., McCormack, B., Seers, K., Tichen, A. (2008) Evaluating the successful implementation of evidence into practice using the PARiHS framework: theoretical and practical challenges. *Implementation Science* **3**. Retrieved 7 February 2008, from www.implementationscience.com/content/3/1/1.

Kjellstrom, T., Norrving, B., Shatchkute, A. (2007) Helsingborg Declaration 2006 on European stroke strategies. *Cerebrovascular Diseases* **23**: 229–241.

LaBresh, K.A.; Paul Coverdell National Acute Stroke Registry. (2006) Quality of acute stroke care improvement framework for the Paul Coverdell National Acute Stroke Registry: facilitating policy and system change at the hospital level. *American Journal of Preventative Medicine* **31**: S246–S250.

Landry, R., Amara, N., Lamari, M. (2002) Does social capital determine innovation? To what extent? *Technological Forecasting and Social Change* **69**: 681–701.

Landry, R., Lyons, R., Amara, N. *et al.* (2006) *Knowledge Translation Planning Tools for Stroke Researchers*. Canadian Stroke Network: Canada.

Lavis, J.N., Ross, S.E., Hurley, J.E. *et al.* (2002) Examining the role of health services research in public policymaking. *The Milbank Quarterly* **80**: 125–154.

Lewis, S. (2007) Can a learning-disabled nation learn healthcare lessons from abroad? *Healthcare Policy* **3**(2): 19–28.

Leys, D., Ringelstein, E.B., Kaste, M., Hacke, W. (2007) Facilities available in European hospitals treating stroke patients. *Stroke* **38**: 2985–2991.

Lyons, R., McGrath, P., Jackson, L., Stone, M. (2005) *The Social Sciences and Humanities in Health Research: A Snapshot of Research Innovation through the Lens of Social Sciences and Humanities*. CIHR/SSHRC: Ottawa.

Lyons, R., McIntyre, L. (July 2007) *The Land of Honey: The New (False) Promise of Prevention*. Presentation at the 19th International Union of Health Promotion and Education, Vancouver, BC.

Lyons, R., Warner, G. (2005) *Demystifying Knowledge Translation for Stroke Researchers: A Primer on Theory and Praxis*. Atlantic Health Promotion Research Centre: Halifax, NS.

Lyons, R., Warner, G., Phillips, S. (2006) Piloting knowledge brokers to enhance health system utilization of stroke research. *A Casebook of Health Services and Policy Research Knowledge Translation Stories*. CIHR: Ottawa.

Matchar, D.B., Samsa, G.P., Sissine, M.E., Howard, G., Warhadpande, D.S. (2007) Promoting the improvement of stroke care at the state level: creating a legislative policy report linked to an evidence-based simulation model. *Value in Health* **10**: 10.

Mayor, S. (2005) Stroke patients prefer care in specialist units. *British Medical Journal* **331**: 130.

Minkman, M., Schouten, L., Huijsman, R., van Splunteren, P. (2005) Integrated care for patients with a stroke in the Netherlands: results and experiences from a national breakthrough collaborative improvement project. *International Journal of Integrated Care* **5**: 1–12.

Mitchell, G.D., Dorling, D., Shaw, M. (2002) Health inequalities in Britain: continuing increases up to the end of the 20th century. *Journal of Epidemiology and Community Health* **6**: 434–435.

National Health Service for Scotland. (2005) *Exploiting the Power of Knowledge in NHS Scotland – a National Strategy*. Retrieved 8 February 2007, from http://www.elib.scot.nhs.uk/news/documents/nhss_knowledge_strategy.pdf.

Nieva, V., Murphy, R., Ridley, N. *et al.* (2005) From science to service: a framework for the transfer of patient safety research into practice. *Advances in Patient Safety* **2**: 441–453.

Pawson, R. (2006) *Evidence-based Policy: A Realist Perspective*. Sage Publications: London.

Petticrew, M., Whitehead, M., MacIntyre, S.J., Graham, H., Egan, M. (2004) Evidence for public health policy on inequalities: 1: the reality according to policymakers. *Journal of Epidemiology and Community Health* **58**: 811–816.

Plochg, T., Klazinga, N. (2002) Community-based integrated care: myth or must? *International Journal for Quality in Health Care* **14**: 91–101.

Prescott, G.L., Lee, R.J., Cohen, G.R. *et al.* (2000) Investigation of factors which might indicate susceptibility to particulate air pollution. *Occupational and Environmental Medicine* **57**: 53–57.

Reich, M.R., Takemi, K., Roberts, M.J., Hsiao, W.O. (2008) Global action on health systems: a proposal for the Tokyo G8 summit. *The Lancet* **371**: 865–869.

Robinson, K., Farmer, T., Riley, B., Elliott, S.J., Eyles, J. (2007) Realistic expectations: investing in organizational capacity building for chronic disease prevention. *American Journal of Health Promotion* **21**: 430–438.

Rogers, E. (1995) *The Diffusion of Innovations*, 4th edition. Free Press: New York.

Rothwell, P. (2007) Making the most of secondary prevention. *Stroke* **38**: 1726.

Sabatier, P. (2007) *Theories of the Policy Process*, 2nd edition. Westview Press: Boulder, CO.

Sabik, L.M., Lie, R. (2008) Priority setting in health care: lessons from the experiences of eight countries. *International Journal for Equity in Health* **7**. Retrieved 10 March 2008, from http://www.pubmedcentral.nih.gov/articlerender.fcgi?artid= 2248188.

Saposnik, G., Kapral, M. (2007) Poststroke care: chronicles of a neglected battle. *Stroke* **38**: 1727–1729.

Schoen, C., Osborn, R., Doty, M., Bishop, M., Peugh, J., Murukutia, N. (2007) Toward higher-performance health systems: adults' health care experiences in seven countries. *Health Affairs* **26**: w717–w734.

Seenan, P., Long, M., Langhorne, P. (2007) Stroke units in their natural habitat: systematic review of observational studies. *Stroke* **38**: 1886–1892.

Singhal, A., Cody, M.J., Rogers, E.M., Sabido, M. (2004) *Entertainment Education and Social Change: History, Research, and Practice*. Lawrence Erlbaum Association: Mahway, NJ.

Stroke Unit Trialists' Collaboration (SUTC). (1997) Collaborative system review of the randomized trials of organized inpatient (stroke unit) care after stroke. *British Medical Journal* **314**: 1151–1158.

Strong, K., Mathers, C., Bonita, R. (2007) Preventing stroke: saving lives around the world. *Lancet* **6**: 182–187.

Truelsen, T., Bonita, R., Jamrozik, K. (2001) Surveillance of stroke: a global perspective. *International Journal of Epidemiology* **30**: S11–S16.

Tugwell, P., Sitthi-Amorn, C., Hatcher-Roberts, J. *et al.* (2006) Health research profile to assess the capacity of low and middle income countries for equity-oriented research. *BMC Public Health* **6**: 151–164.

U.S. Census Bureau. (2003) *Characteristics of the Civilian Non-institutionalized Population by Age, Disability Status, and Type of Disability 2000*.

Watkins, P. (2004) Chronic disease. *Clinical Medicine* **4**: 297–298.

Weinstein, M.C., Toy, E.L., Sandberg, E.A. *et al.* (2001) Modeling of health care and other policy decisions: uses, roles and validity. *Value in Health* **4**: 348–361.

Wentworth, D.A., Atkinson, R.P. (1996) Implementation of an acute stroke program decreases hospitalization costs and length of stay. *Stroke* **27**: 1040–1043.

Whitfield, M.D., Gillett, M., Holmes, M., Ogden, E. (2006) Predicting the impact of population level risk reduction in cardio-vascular disease and stroke on acute hospital admission rates over a 5 year period – a pilot study. *Public Health* **120**: 1140–1148.

Wolfe, C., Rudd, A.G., McKevitt, C., Heuschmann, P., Kalra, L. (2007) *Development of a European Implementation Score for Measuring Implementation of Research into Healthcare Practice Using Vascular Disease as an Example*. Research proposal to the European Union. Retrieved 20 March 2008 from http://www.kcl.ac.uk/schools/medicine/research/hscr/eis.html.

Woods, K. (2001) The development of integrated health care models in Scotland. *International Journal of Integrated Care* **1**: 1–16.

Woolf, S.H. (8 January 2006) Unhealthy medicine: all breakthrough, no follow through. *Washington Post.* Retrieved 10 January 2008, from http://www.washingtonpost.com/wp-.

World Health Organization. (2008) *World Health Statistics 2008.* www.who.in./statistics (accessed in 2008).

Yach, D., Leeder, S.R., Bell, J., Kistnasamy, B. (2005) Global chronic disease. *Science* **307**: 317.

Zhang, N., Wu, A., Weller, W., Anderson, G. (2001) *National Health Care Expenditures Projections, 2000–2010.*

9. *Future Directions*

Debbie Kralik

The authors of the innovative chapters in this book have articulated new ways of conceptualising chronic illness research and demonstrated the translation of that knowledge into clinical practice. They have identified future challenges and opportunities for chronic illness research and practice. The broad challenges, on a global scale, are how we can

- prevent, delay, detect and control chronic diseases across one's lifespan;
- apply research to put practical and effective intervention strategies into practice;
- realise equity in health by eliminating racial and ethnic disparities and achieving optimal health for all populations.

Underpinning each of these broad challenges is effective knowledge translation. The authors of Chapter 8 articulate very clearly the barriers and enablers of knowledge translation. Translation is profoundly important if we are to make any difference to chronic illness prevention, treatment and care. Translation of chronic illness research into practice is dependent on how informed and receptive policymakers, health professionals, health organisations and consumers are to innovation.

The need for such significant change and the development of solutions that facilitate the uptake of research into practice continues to challenge researchers and practitioners. While there is a wealth of knowledge available about chronic diseases and chronic illness experience, there is significant debate about the impact of that knowledge on policy and practice. The authors of this book have highlighted the need not only for research initiatives but also for developing strategies that will facilitate the implementation of research into practice settings where consumers can benefit. In this concluding chapter, we revisit some of the issues raised in the body of this book for further discussion and consider future directions for chronic illness research.

Global perspective

The broad impact of globalisation on chronic illness research was explored in Chapter 1. Globalisation is the increasing interconnectedness of countries, and the opening of borders to ideas, people, commerce and finances has had both beneficial and harmful effects on the health of populations (Beaglehole & Yach 2003). Health is impacted upon by broader issues and complexities such as globalisation, quality housing, changes in nutritional norms, access to education, information technology explosion, unhealthy environments, global warming, multiculturalism and the central place of health care in global politics. We cannot ignore these phenomena if we are to truly shape chronic illness health care. It is of global importance that we pay attention because no country will have the resources to provide in totality the chronic illness health-care needs and wants of its communities. The World Health Organization (WHO) and governments alone are increasingly unable to address the breadth of control challenges related to the escalation of chronic diseases. Local resources such as informal carers, equipment, qualified professionals and finances needed for the management of chronic diseases always have a limit. The challenge is to develop through research, new and innovative models of care and health promotion, which influence both the prevalence of chronic disease and the effectiveness of health services for people living with chronic conditions.

The WHO has established strategies and programmes to impact areas such as physical activity and nutrition, reducing tobacco smoking and alcohol consumption, but the reality is that the translation of these strategies needs to occur at a local level. A major issue is that there exist considerable differences in research funding, resources and infrastructure that support chronic illness management in different countries and regions. Such diversity impacts the initiatives being implemented and evaluated on an international scale. Given these challenges, chronic illness researchers will need to find ways of being active on a global level, by establishing strong international networks, conducting international studies and being committed to publication.

Facilitating the will of the people

Responding to the global burden of chronic conditions requires strategic vision, political will, assessment, implementation and evaluation of the processes most likely to encourage policy change (Magnusson 2007). The major mechanism of policy change that will positively impact people with chronic illness is public will – that is, the emergence and escalation of the agendas, priorities and values of consumers shaping policy through local area engagement activities. This is where researchers, health practitioners and consumers can work collaboratively to demonstrate political awareness with a view to changing local policy that will promote implementation of chronic illness health-care initiatives. We need to think globally, but collaborate with consumers to act locally using the best evidence available as indicators of effective care intervention. Processes for encouraging local consumer participation may be considered to be in their infancy, but as demonstrated by the examples cited in this book, organisations are exploring ways of ensuring genuine consumer involvement, and legitimate partnerships are fostered. Generating public will through genuine consumer involvement is central to increasing the effectiveness of chronic illness research and health care in the future. Greater consumer involvement will have the added benefit of promoting health literacy, enhancing consumer capacity to self-care, and raising the level of broader community awareness about chronic illness and preventative actions. The sustainability of future health systems depends on consumer involvement.

The evidence base

Highlighted by several examples cited in this book is that we continue to draw much of our learning from research conducted in large metropolitan centres in predominantly developed countries. There are many more initiatives that could serve as indicators for the future development of chronic disease prevention and management, but these are not widely publicised and there is a decided lack of empirical evidence and evaluation to support their adoption in other settings. Each of us working in the area of chronic illness care and research will know of many examples of projects that are locally driven and focus on the management, early intervention and prevention of a chronic disease of interest to the local community. Unfortunately, we rarely hear about the effectiveness of these programmes either because they are not sustained or because they are continued without evaluation (Wakerman *et al.* 2005). Considerable time and resource is required to increase knowledge, translate it into practice with the associated behavioural change and then measure change in health indicators such as clinical outcomes (Wakerman *et al.* 2005). Many research projects, particularly those involving people in rural and remote communities and with marginalised populations, are often not afforded this time or resources and therefore have little capacity to influence policy development.

Crucial to the further development of chronic illness research is a clear under-standing of the broad research base that extends across disciplines. Many of the initiatives cited in this book may not be known to health-care practitioners who confine their reading of research-based evidence to journals and texts in their own language, discipline or nation. A broadening of our strategies for communicating and knowledge sharing is vital for successful translation of chronic illness research in the future.

Technology and health promotion

Health promotion is critical for the prevention of chronic diseases. A variety of health communication strategies are used in health promotion to deliver culturally appropriate and effective health-related messages. These interven-tions include paid advertising, media advocacy, public relations, health pro-motion activities and campaigns that target specific audiences. These health promotion activities will continue to increase and utilise new and emerging tech-nologies and communication strategies such as Twitter. The future will see technology and interactive telecommunications assisting in the translation of chronic illness research into practice. The dramatic advances in computing and communication technologies mean that researchers, policymakers, practitioners and consumers have greater access to knowledge and information about trends in chronic disease, clinical indicators and outcome measures about treatments and inform health promotion messages. Technology will continue to grow and impact the point of clinical care, providing clinicians with real time data upon which to base decisions. The major obstruction to the uptake of these technologies, however, has been the resistance of health-care professionals to implement it in practice (Cooke *et al.* 2009). This is thought to be because fundamental changes to clinical practice are required to support tele-health technologies. Another challenge is the disparity in access to these technologies across socio-economic groups. Based on previous trends, however, the proportion of people using these technologies will continue to increase, which will narrow the current divide.

Transition

Chapter 2 explored the construct of transition and in so doing highlighted the disparity in the published qualitative literature regarding the experience of living with chronic illness. Learning to live with chronic illness is an ongoing complex and personal process that can occur over a long period of time. The chronic illness experience has been described in many ways including as a trajectory, a gift, a career, a dichotomy between acceptance and denial, transformation and as the cause of feelings of chronic sorrow, suffering, uncertainty and loss. The chronic illness experience may include all of these understandings; so how have such variations in interpretation come about? Perhaps the dearth of longitudinal studies about chronic illness experience has resulted in chronic illness research highlighting 'snap shots' of people's experiences of living with chronic illness. Most studies present a person's position at a particular point in time, so we may lack the full picture that informs us of the breadth of that experience over time. Consequently, the literature results in differing interpretations of the chronic illness experience.

Living with chronic illness is an ever-changing experience. Chronic illness can take many forms and there is no single pattern of experience even within the same diagnosis. Considerable adjustment and adaptation to daily life is required to incorporate the symptoms and consequences of illness. The process of learning to live with chronic illness involves the need for transition, requiring people to adjust and modify their responses, behaviours and attitudes to ever-changing life situations. A major limitation of much of the published chronic illness research is its short-term focus. The passage of time can be a militating or mitigating factor in transition. As such, longitudinal studies are required to explore experiences that promote transition. Further research is required to enhance our understanding of what services will assist people living with chronic illness through the phases of transition. Gaps in transition research relate to gendered responses to change events, the transitional experiences during an acute episode of illness, the differences in transition across the lifespan and the specific interventions/activities that facilitate transition during the various trajectories of chronic illness.

Self-management and self-care

Self-care and self-management are terms that have often been used interchangeably in the literature, although we are learning that they do not have the same meaning. Self-management has been consistently advocated as a way of containing the impact of chronic disease through health workers and client working in partnership. Self-care is the ability of the person to adapt to the changes that are taking place in his or her life because of illness and to learn ways to deal with all that living with chronic illness entails, including symptoms, treatment, physical and social consequences and lifestyle changes and disruption. The focus of self-care recognises that the persons themselves are the principle caregivers and decision makers.

Self-care decisions are informed by the personal and social context of people's lives. Medical or health advice may not always be prioritised. A type of wisdom evolves from the long-term experience of living day-to-day with a chronic illness. This involves being faced with vital dilemmas caused by changing responses to being in the world. The person faces this alone since health professionals and others are not there in everyday life situations. The process of searching for options, trialling actions and activities and experiencing the consequences equips persons with a depth of knowledge about how their body responds in certain situations. People make self-care decisions against a background of complex sociocultural characteristics, psychological interpretations, spiritual beliefs and personal priorities. Consequently, the nature of self-care will be unique to the person and will change over time and circumstances. Making a decision to self-care does not guarantee that this will always be the way the person approaches living with illness. Just as chronic illness is influenced by the wider context of people's lives so too is the willingness and ability to be involved in self-care decisions. Cultural norms, values and beliefs inform both people's attitudes to self-care and the shape it takes. There is much research to be undertaken in this area. Future directions involve building upon the existing evidence so that we may move towards targeted and effective self-management interventions that enhance the capacity of people with chronic illness to self-care.

Health in the community

Most health care for people with chronic disease occurs in the community setting in the context of their daily lives. Comprehensive knowledge and understanding of the context in which the person lives, family, carers, supporters, community and wider society form an important backdrop to successful chronic disease health care. People with one chronic disease often develop multiple illnesses, which are referred to as *co-morbidities* as discussed in Chapter 4. This adds another layer of complexity to a health system that is largely framed by a single disease model of care. Much research has been disease or symptom specific; hence research is needed that will assist in the understanding of the impact of disease co-morbidity on individuals and communities. While there has been significant progress made in the clinical management of common chronic diseases, much less is known about the impact of co-morbidity, including physical and mental health co-morbidities, on disease management, clinical outcomes, quality of life and quality improvements.

The effective elements of a community health-care system that promotes high-quality chronic disease care are population profiling of the community, development of processes that articulate community needs, consumer participation, person-centred care, self-management support, decision support and clinical information systems and an emphasis on building effective multidisciplinary teams. Within this context, evidence-based change concepts will further foster productive interactions between informed people in our communities, who take an active part in their care, and multidisciplinary providers with resources and expertise. Future research needs to focus on systems that integrate preventative, acute and chronic co-morbidity, rehabilitative and long-term care focused on reducing illness burden and improving health-related quality of life. Given the increasing prevalence of chronic illness and the aging population, research is needed that will reduce the economic and social burden of chronic disease, arrest or slow deterioration, and prevent disability from these illnesses.

These will be the paramount issues in public health for the foreseeable future.

References

Beaglehole, R., Yach, D. (2003) Globalisation and the prevention and control of non-communicable disease: the neglected chronic diseases of adults. *The Lancet* **362** (9387): 903–908.

Cooke, D., Sheetal, P., Newman, S. (2009) Facilitating self-management through telemedicine and interactive health communication applications. In: Newman, S., Steed, L., Mulligan, K. (eds) *Chronic Physical Illness: Self Management and Behavioural Interventions*. Open University Press: Berkshire.

Magnusson, R. (2007) Non-communicable diseases and global health governance: enhancing global processes to improve health development. *Globalization and Health* **3**: 2.

Wakerman, J., Chalmers, E., Humphreys, J. *et al.* (2005) Sustainable chronic disease management in remote Australia. *Medical Journal of Australia* **183**(10): s64–s68.

Index